Women Living with Multiple Sclerosis

What others are saying . . .

". . . [E]ngaging both as a description of the uses of a powerful new technology for sharing information and experience, and as an argument for the benefits of support groups as vehicles of human caring . . . several chapters are particularly interesting. The discussion of sex, for example, was one of the best I've ever come across in its factual content, honesty, delicacy, and humor. I can envision readers sharing selected passages from the book with family or friends to facilitate more open communication.

The book is a validation of experience for those who have been in support groups, an invitation to those who have not yet done so, and a celebration of the wonder and pleasure that these particular women take in having found each other."
— Anne-Elizabeth Straub, CSW, *Inside MS*

"What makes this book different from other medical books is that many of these topics rarely are discussed in the doctor's office, usually because of embarrassment [and] hesitancy . . ."
— *The Cincinnati Enquirer*

"Recommended for all general collections and caregivers and physicians involved with MS patients."
— *Library Journal*

Women Living with Multiple Sclerosis

Judith Lynn Nichols
and Her Group of Online MS Sisters

Hunter House Inc., Publishers
P.O. Box 2914
Alameda CA 94501-0914

Library of Congress Cataloging-in-Publication Data
Nichols, Judith Lynn
Women living with multiple sclerosis / Judith Lynn Nichols.
p. cm.
Includes index.
ISBN 0-89793-218-8
1. Multiple Sclerosis—Popular works. 2. Women—Diseases. I. Title.
RC377.N53 1999
362.1'96834'0082—dc21 98-35659
CIP

Project credits

Cover Design: MIG Communications   Book Design: *Qalagraphia*
Commissioning Editor: Kiran S. Rana   Production Coordinator: Wendy Low
Editor: Laura Harger   Proofreader: Lee Rappold
Promotion: Marisa Spatafore   Marketing Intern: Monique Portegies
Editorial Assistants: Jennifer Rader, Jeanne Brondino
Customer Support: Christina Arciniega, Joel Irons
Order fulfillment: A & A Quality Shipping Services
Publisher: Kiran S. Rana

Printed and Bound by Publishers Press, Salt Lake City, UT
Manufactured in the United States of America

9 8 7 6 5 4   First Edition   00 01 02 03 04

Table of Contents

Dedicated to:

Ron and Karen and Julie,
for loving me in sickness and in health.

The Flutterbuds, for flying with me.

Acknowledgments

I'm just beginning to realize how many people contributed in some way to the creation of this book. I'm grateful to each of them. Special thanks to:

... my husband, Ron Nichols, who provided, in addition to his constant faith and love, everything from voice recognition software when I couldn't type to dinners when I was too busy to cook;

... the people at Hunter House, especially Kiran Rana, who led me to my launching pad;

... my editor, Laura Harger, who gently turned over each word to make sure it fit. Now I know why authors thank their editors;

... the ladies in the Froup, who satisfied my obsession; and their loved ones, who let me share their family secrets;

... Brenda and Patti and Reva, who couldn't lend their names but offered their words and their spirit;

... Karen Heyl, who made me believe this day would come;

... Nancy Scgan, who has been my "first editor" for more than thirty-five years;

... my cheering section: Donna Gabbard, Sis Thomas, Nell Stone, Sandie Tieman, Joyce Kiefer, Ruth Bell, Sandy Howard, Jean Hoffman, and, of course, Karen and Julie Nichols;

... my God, who engineered this project and gave me everything I needed at the exact moment I needed it.

Foreword

by Robert L. Reed, M.D.

I read this book with tremendous enthusiasm. The remarkable medium of the Internet allowed more than twenty women with MS to share their most personal experiences; indeed, there may be no other communications medium which enables such frank disclosure. The authenticity of the women and their experiences make this book, in my view, truly unique.

The two messages from this book that hit home with the greatest impact for me are that the caregiver who fails to listen does a great disservice to his or her patients; and that for the patient, to be heard and to share experiences is mandatory for the healing process to begin. Getting better is not always the same as healing.

As a neurologist, I have been caring for people with multiple sclerosis for twenty-five years, but until reading this book I never fully understood the depth of suffering the patient with MS endures. For example, the frankness of the chapter "And Then There's Sex . . . !" opened my mind to a whole new set of problems I did not fully appreciate. This chapter alone suggests many areas in which my staff and I can help, and I plan to begin doing so right away. Because it is obvious from the book that many women prefer to avoid discussing the subject of sex with male physicians, I have asked one of my medical assistants—a warm and sensitive communicator—to read the chapter, and become the person to broach the subject of sexuality with our women MS patients.

Doctors and others in the medical field need to learn how we can do a better job for our patients. The first half of this book is a strong indictment of the physician who is incapable of dealing with a patient with a disease of the complexity of MS (as well as other disabling diseases). I think most of us physicians will see ourselves in the various doctors described in this book and blush with shame. In our frustration, we may turn to cruel tactics that drive our patients away. Out of sight, not my problem. We need input such as that found in *Women Living with Multiple Sclerosis* to learn how we can help patients deal with more than just the medical management of their disease.

This book must also serve as an inspiration to all who may view their productive lives as shortened by disabilities such as multiple sclerosis. Judy Nichols' first love has always been writing, and MS has not blunted her talent or desire. I personally commend her for such a fine effort, and will recommend this book to each and every one of my patients with MS.

— Robert M. Reed, M.D.,
Riverhills Healthcare Neurology Division,
Cincinnati, Ohio

Preface

For all of my adult life (and that's much more than half of my entire life!), I've lived with a monster. For all of those years, I've fought to survive its assaults and to keep body, mind, and spirit integrated and intact. I've struggled to preserve some modicum of peace in my family, aware that at any moment my assailant might turn up, might in an instant demolish once more everything that we've worked so hard to rebuild and maintain since its last appearance.

For most of those years, I thought my conflict was effectively a solitary one. I knew that somewhere there were others, especially other women, who wrestled with the same demon. But I'd never made contact with these fellow combatants, at least not in a way that permitted me to know them well enough that we could care for one another as people, rather than merely as fellow sufferers of multiple sclerosis.

Then, within a very short time last year, I met and became friends with more than twenty of these similar souls, all of whom wage their own war against the Beast. Since then, we've learned with one another and from one another ways to best use the defenses available to us. We've shared the means we've discovered to let us move on in our lives with some measure of dignity, some serenity of spirit, some remission from pain, loneliness, frustration, and misery. We've helped one another to endure the unendurable, even to find humor, at times, in our forced associations with our captor.

We're not the harem of an abusive master or a support group for battered wives. We're just ordinary women who each happen to need information, support, companionship, and dialogue with others who can really share what goes on in our daily battles with the common adversary we carry within our bodies. We all have multiple sclerosis.

We met in the MS information area of an Internet server. After some months of getting to know one another, it became clear that some of the participants there had discovered a special connection. We sought a more relaxed, intimate atmosphere than was possible in the board's public arena. A handful of "board members," including myself, began to communicate more closely among ourselves, and then we invited still others to add their opinions and tell us about their experiences. Before long, we found that each of us was reaching out consistently to the same twenty-plus names on our mailing lists. Thus, our group—now known as the "Froup," or the Flutterbuds' Group, named for the mental "flutters" that sometimes plague MSers—was born. (For more information on how the "Froup" formed, and some advice on forming your own online group, see the Resources section at the end of the book.)

We correspond daily by means of round-robin online letters to all the other members on our common mailing list. We talk about everything related to coping with life with our chronic, progressive disease. After a while, the Froup and I realized that our discussions would be of interest to others who are coping with life with the MS monster, and the idea for this book was born. Because most of our MS-related discussions started on the Internet message boards, each of which is dedicated to a specific aspect of life with MS, I kept that same form for the book—each chapter picks up and continues one of the dialogues that we began online, touching on topics from diagnosis to family life to sexuality to work. Sometimes, of course, we talk about much that is unrelated to any disease at all. We haven't included those conversations here. They're best saved for another book.

Some of what is contained in this book is lifted, with the authors' permission, directly from the message-board conversations. Other entries were E-mailed to me as part of our round-robin coffee klatches or in response to my request for submissions. Occasionally, if I was aware that a member had a particular interest in a topic that I wanted to write about, I asked for her thoughts on that topic. Always, though, my request was copied to all members, and the respondents' answers were likewise circulated to all. That way, anybody was welcome to jump into the discussion and add her two cents worth. This also helped to solidify the immense group friendship that has grown out of our association. It has given each of us equal opportunity to know the others.

Out of respect for those who prefer to maintain the anonymous nature of the Internet, I've changed the screen names and other identifying characteristics of all authors except those who gave me express permission to use them as originally written.

This book is a narrative of day-to-day life with multiple sclerosis. It's meant to illustrate what life with this monster entails, to show what modifications have had to be adopted, then changed and re-adopted again and again to satisfy the appetites of the Beast. We hope that allowing others, MSers or just interested people, to read about our experiences will give them some idea of the agony and the ecstasy inherent in our individual lives and in the collective life that has evolved for us online.

Meet the MonSter

To understand the intensity and the diversity of the struggles that people with MS encounter every day, it's useful to first look at some medical facts, beginning with a description of multiple sclerosis from a clinical perspective.

MS is a disease of the central nervous system, including the brain and spinal cord. The brain is supposed to send signals, via the spinal cord and an intricate system of nerves, to all parts of the body. The signals let the body parts know what they're supposed to do at any particular time (move, relax, react to outside stimuli such as pain or heat, etc.). This whole system is protected by a fatty covering called the myelin sheath. When multiple sclerosis comes along, it tricks the body's immune system into attacking the myelin covering, breaking it down in patchy areas throughout the system. This causes the formation of sclerotic (hardened) spots, which get in the way of the brain's messages, distorting them or blocking them entirely. As a result, the feet can't walk, the hands can't touch, the eyes can't see. Malfunctions can occur in just about any part of the anatomy, depending on what area of the nervous system is currently affected.

MS carries with it a mixed bag of tricks, which it distributes to its captives at random in the form of varied symptoms. These can include numbness, tingling, and other strange sensory perceptions, such as buzzing or crawling or burning sensations on the skin, for which there's no apparent reason. There might be motor problems, such as the inability to walk, raise an arm, grasp, or hold onto something; these can eventually progress to paralysis. There can be a general experience of "klutziness," imbalance or uncoordination. Vision or hearing may be impaired, suddenly or gradually. There may be difficulty in controlling the eye muscles, so focus is off or vision is double or "jumpy." There can be muscle spasms anywhere in the body, difficulty speaking, difficulty swallowing. Problems with bladder control are common, with episodes of retention or incontinence. The same is true of bowel control. There might be emotional upsets, pain, overwhelming fatigue.

Most MSers never have all these symptoms at once, or even at different times. Some go through a whole lifetime with nothing more than a couple of mild episodes that cause problems only in very limited areas.

It's impossible to predict the course of the disease in any individual. The MonSter likes to make its first appearance when its victim is between the ages of twenty and forty, although some cases have been diagnosed before age ten or after age fifty. At first, the condition generally involves attacks, or exacerbations, in which symptoms last from a few hours to several months. Then a period of remission occurs, during which the patient seems to recover, sometimes with no obvious residual effects. Experts say this occurs because the myelin is capable of repairing itself, at least for a while. The hiatus may last months, even years, before a new attack sets in. Sometimes this pattern of relapse and recovery continues indefinitely (this kind of MS is known as the relapsing/remitting type). In many people, the remissions eventually become less frequent and are less complete; attacks are less defined, and steadily increasing disability ensues (this is known as the secondary progressive type). In other cases, there aren't any real remissions; the disease progresses steadily from the onset, with perhaps an occasional "plateau" time when everything seems to remain stable for a while (primary progressive type). For some, finally, the MS progresses consistently, with no remissions or plateaus, but with occasional times of dramatic attacks or worsening symptoms (progressive relapsing type).

Fortunately, those who go steadily downhill are in the minority. It should be remembered, too, that when it comes to MS, very few firm pronouncements are allowed. There can occasionally be crossovers between two or more types, so that a patient may start out in one classification, switch to another, and then move to another or back to the original.

People with MS usually don't die from it. In the most severe cases, which make up only a very small percentage of the overall MS population, there might be complications such as pneumonia, severe urinary tract infections, and skin breakdown that are potentially fatal, but MS itself rarely causes death. The life expectancy for MSers is close to that for people without MS. More than a third of a million people in the United States have been diagnosed with multiple sclerosis; many more cases may remain undiagnosed because MS's symptoms sometimes mimic those of other conditions. Multiple sclerosis isn't contagious, and it isn't inherited, although familial susceptibility to the condition is sometimes apparent.

At the present time, there's no known cure for MS. So there's nothing to be done about it, at least as far as stopping it completely is concerned. There are, however, several very effective treatments now available that may lessen the frequency and severity of attacks, reduce the risk of permanent damage, and minimize existing symptoms. And it seems that there's always word of still another new drug or treatment being tested against MS.

Probably the most common treatment is intravenous steroid infusions, administered over a period of several days. This is usually done at the beginning of an exacerbation as a means of reducing inflammation and preventing permanent trauma to the nervous system. The bad news about such treatment is that it usually involves a number of side effects. These can include water retention, weight gain, increased susceptibility to infection, loss of bone mass, insomnia, and mental changes. Side effects seem most obvious just after the patient finishes the course of treatment. Until the medication leaves the system completely, he or she is usually plagued by the above effects, accompanied by a period of hyperactivity that isn't relieved by sleeping pills or other sedative measures. The ladies in our group usually refer to this time as "doing the steroid shuffle."

The good news is that this same period is frequently marked by a most welcome mental change, a feeling of well-being that can extend to pure euphoria. Sometimes, too, the hyperactivity results in clean houses, caught-up paperwork, completion of all the tasks that usually have to compete for attention with MS's gift of chronic fatigue. The best news is that these treatments can effect a dramatic improvement in the patient's condition, at least temporarily.

For the past few years, many people with MS have been able to slow the progress of the disease by using one of the interferons or copolymers. There can be side effects with these, too, usually flu-like symptoms that subside after the body adjusts to the presence of the medication. I used an interferon for more than a year. I gave myself an injection every other day; the thought of doing it was scary at first, but it soon became as routine as taking a pill. And it did slow the progress of my symptoms for that year. I'd probably still be on it, but eventually I developed a hypersensitivity to the drug, which caused me to break out in hives.

I'm now taking an immunosuppressant in an effort to keep the immune system from attacking itself. This is considered a rather radical treatment; I don't personally know another MSer on the same medication. My neurologist warned me at the beginning that this drug would lower my resistance to infection to a possibly dangerous level. He also advised that eventually the drug could cause cancer of the lymphatic system. He suggested that I ask the hematologist/oncologist I was seeing at the time for his opinion. This doctor said, "Your neurological condition is deteriorating every day.

Look at it this way: Use the medication and you might have five more years of a full, productive life. Don't use it, and you might live for ten more years, but you'll have continually increasing disability, to the point where you really won't be living at all." It didn't take much more than that to convince me to start the treatment.

So far, I've been happy with the results. For almost a full year, my symptoms remained stable. It's only recently that there has been further progression. My blood is checked at least once a month to keep track of any changes. Nothing alarming has shown up during this time.

Aside from these few systemic remedies, multiple sclerosis is usually treated symptomatically. Each of the ladies in our group takes an assortment of muscle relaxers, painkillers, antidepressants, and, frequently, nutritional supplements. Sharon, for example, tells us that she couldn't get along without her "megadoses" of vitamins and supplements. (Sharon has done extensive research into this treatment, has had professional assessment of her needs based on many factors in addition to her MS, and takes the vitamins and supplements under professional guidance. She recommends that anyone considering such therapy do the same.) Some of us manage or minimize symptoms through exercise programs, physical or occupational therapy, meditation, and relaxation techniques.

We understand that further advancements in finding treatments and a cure for MS will be expedited by determining what cave this MonSter crawled out of. Ongoing research is trying to find out how it came into being, and how it got from there and then to here and now. Much of the research shows that there is a virus involved somewhere, but nobody knows exactly which virus or what role it plays. One theory suggests that one or more viruses, introduced into a person's system during childhood, remain dormant for years until some other factor (genetic? environmental?) triggers them to become active again. Then, experts say, some kind of mix-up in the immune system causes it to confuse the virus with myelin and to begin to destroy the myelin.

There have been any number of theories as to what triggers this mix-up. Investigation has been done into trauma, hormone imbalance, exposure to some toxin or another, suppression of sweat, and poor blood circulation, to name just a few. So far, there is no proof that any of these factors has a direct relation to MS. The research continues, but for now the answer to "What causes MS?" is still a big "Who knows?"

Have you noticed that almost every statement about multiple sclerosis is preceded by an indefinite term such as *usually, almost always, sometimes, may, can, might?* That's because the only thing that's consistent about MS is its inconsistency from one individual to another, and also within each individual. Symptoms and progression vary from person to person, and it's difficult to predict the disease's path in any patient with any accuracy. With multiple sclerosis, the only thing we can count on is that we can't count on anything. That's not all bad. It means that for people with MS, forever doesn't always mean always. There have been patients whose severely disabling MS somehow "burned out," leaving no long-term effects. There's always the chance that this will happen for each and every one of us. Meanwhile, we just go on living with the MonSter. That's what all the conversations in this book are about.

2

Cast of Characters

Meet the Flutterbuds, the "characters" who so generously and honestly shared with me their stories about life with multiple sclerosis, and then agreed that we could share their stories with everybody who reads this book.

▲▲▲

RENEE is forty-five. She and her husband, Burt, have six children/stepchildren and are raising their grandson Dominic, who is ten. Officially diagnosed in 1986, she uses a cane for balance and support. She has frequent problems with vision, cognitive function, and sensory perception in her extremities.

We call Renee "Cybermom" because, besides being the chief founding member of our Froup, she has assumed a kind of maternal responsibility for each of our members. She's also "Queen of Purple Gak." Any time a member of our group encounters a major life change, whether good or bad, Renee throws a handful of a sticky, slimy substance known as Gak at a designated space on one of the walls in her home (reserved just for this purpose). "Gakking" a person is the symbolic equivalent of a prayer, a blessing, a celebration, or a sympathetic gesture, as fits the occasion.

▲▲▲

JANE, forty-eight, was diagnosed with multiple sclerosis as a twenty-four-year-old newlywed, when she lost the vision in one eye (the vision returned several weeks later after treatment with adreno-corticotrophic hormone, or ACTH). "It's only during the past six months that I've had four more episodes of temporary blindness— a pretty good record for twenty-four years of living with MS!"

Married and the mother of three almost-adult children, Jane leads a weekly online worship service for people with multiple sclerosis and is involved in four weekly online support groups.

There are seldom two days in a row when I don't see that God has led me to someone or someone to me. It is awesome to see him so active in cyberspace, which, of course, he is, in a big way!

Jane uses "Tingles" as her online signature.

▲▲▲

LORI, twenty-eight, is married to Steve and has a young daughter, Amanda. She began having symptoms of multiple sclerosis when she was seventeen or eighteen years old. She didn't start to actively search for a diagnosis until the past year. She has official diagnoses of fibromyalgia, intention tremor, and neurogenic bladder (see the glossary). Her doctors believe that her symptoms and abnormal neurological exams make it "highly probable" that she has MS; they have not given her a firm diagnosis so far.

She is currently ambulatory and uses a cane for balance. Her most troublesome symptoms are fatigue, cognitive issues, pain, tremors, and migraines ("which may or may not be related to the multiple sclerosis").

Lori worked as an executive secretary for the president/CEO of a large development firm until December of 1996. At that time, stress-induced fatigue and many other symptoms played a large role in her decision to adopt a more sedate lifestyle.

Before all of this started to affect me physically, I was very active. I used to love to rappel and mountain climb and was active in the MP unit of the Army National Guard. I am having a hard time getting to the point where I am thankful for actually getting to do some of the things I used to do, instead of being resentful that I am no longer able to do all of them. I get a little bit farther every day, though.

The baby of the Froup, Lori is nicknamed "Whippersnapper."

▲▲▲

JANIS, forty-two, is married, with two young children. She is still in the remitting/relapsing stage of multiple sclerosis, and she seems to do a lot of both. We call her "Rainbow" because she looks for one in every dark situation.

I am a fighter, and I will not let this disease get the best of me, no matter what it throws at me.

▲▲▲

CHRIS, forty-five, is married, and has a twenty-year-old son. She was diagnosed in 1995, and her current condition involves "lots of cognitive problems, which sometimes make life a real challenge!!!"

She recently began to use a cane for walking, which she considers another challenge. Other symptoms include fatigue, vision problems, "and the list goes on and on!!!"

Chris is nicknamed "MS Excited," because of her liberal use of exclamation marks when she "talks" online.

▲▲▲

BREN is thirty-four years old. She lives with Al, her significant other, and has two daughters. Diagnosed in 1993, she can trace MS symptoms back as far as 1984. She is currently ambulatory and uses no aids (such as a cane or wheelchair. Most of her symptoms are related to fatigue and cognitive function. Her physical problems are mild so far, with some numbness and weakness in her limbs.

Bren is the jokester of the group.

I love to hear folks laugh and to make them smile. I have the nickname "Wicked Ms. Fixit." That came about when Renee was feeling very bad after a bout with I.V. steroid treatment. I wrote her a soothing letter and talked her through some meditation to help her relax. She dubbed me "Ms. Fixit." Soon afterward, someone else said she always imagined me with not just a grin, but a wicked grin. Hence "Wicked Ms. Fixit." I really do like to fix things. I carry a mean toolbelt, when I can find the dang thing. I keep forgetting to get it out of Sally's Fridge . . . [See Chapter Four].

▲▲▲

RAMIA was diagnosed in 1997 at the age of thirty-eight. We call her "Momia Ramia" (her choice) because she is heavily involved (also her choice) with her and her husband's two children, ages six and two.

▲▲▲

KIM, thirty-seven, is single and lives with her father and brother. So far, the MS has caused her to walk with a limp. She has experienced minor cognitive changes and "weird feelings." She also has significant problems with bladder control. "My eyes are still terrific, though, I am happy to say!"

Kim is a nurse and works with Alzheimer's patients. She is nicknamed "Tinkerbell" because of the hypothetical pouch of fairy dust she carries around to sprinkle on all of us who need some magic in our lives.

▲▲▲

HELEN is fifty-six. She lives with her housemate, Janni, and has a nineteen-year-old foster son. She was diagnosed about eight years ago but says that she has "had this damned disease forever, but got brushed aside by doctors for far too many years."

I seem to have mild chronic-progressive MS, since when I exacerbate, the damned symptoms don't ALL go away afterward. I'm blind in my left eye, have motor control problems with my hands, and walk with a limp. Other than that, I look so good (for being short and fat with dyed hair).

Helen nicknamed herself "Curmudgeon," although the rest of us have questioned the validity of the label. She explains:

When I get down in the dumps or frustrated, I get really bitchy. "Curmudgeon" sounds better than "Bitch," don't you think? I'm a skeptic and a pessimist, and if I didn't have a sense of humor to balance it all out, I'd be a total pain in the ass.

▲▲▲

PAT, forty-nine, is married, with two children. She was diagnosed in 1977 but feels that the MonSter has always been a part of her life. She's ambulatory but uses crutches or a wheelchair when necessary. Her symptoms are sensory, visual, "and much more; let us not forget bladder and bowel problems, shall we?"

Pat's nickname is "Angel Mom." She got that when she added to one of her letters a plea to God to send her an angel to help her through a bad time. Then she amended it to acknowledge that he'd already sent her a whole bunch of "angels" in the form of our group.

▲▲▲

SHARON, forty-six, was diagnosed in 1994. She is still relapsing/remitting and ambulatory without aids. She is engaged to Bob and has four teens.

Sharon has dubbed herself "Yankee Princess" ("I just love to ruffle the feathers of the Southern belles in the Froup"). We also know her as "Psych Lady." A practicing therapist, she prefers to keep her work separate from her participation in our group. We do, however, ask for and receive her professional input on many subjects.

▲▲▲

DEE, fifty-four, is happily married, with a blended family of fourteen children and an "army" of grandchildren and great-grandchildren.

After many months of testing and diagnoses of fibromyalgia, arthritis, vestibular disorder, and vision disorders, her doctors have only recently concluded that she has MS. Dee describes herself as currently "ambulatory, but unsteady, vision-impaired, and dizzy. (I've always been dizzy, I know.)"

Dee has nicknamed herself "Dee-Duh." We don't know if she's singing or talking about her affinity for the mental flutters, or confusion, that often accompany MS.

▲▲▲

JAMIE was diagnosed with chronic progressive MS when she was twenty-three. At one point, she wasn't expected to live through that first crisis. She defied predictions, though, and made an amazing comeback. Now, at thirty-five, she's fairly stable and uses a cane and wheelchair as necessary. She is blind in one eye and has limited vision in the other, the result of her first battle with the MonSter. Her significant other is Jeff, and she has one daughter, Jaylon, "my miracle child, born two years after my diagnosis."

Jamie's nickname is "Biker Babe" because she loves Harleys and still rides every chance she gets. "I can't drive because I can't see and can't walk without aid, but put me on a Harley and I'm fine!"

▲▲▲

TARA, forty-two, is the divorced mother of three young-adult sons. She had a possible/probable diagnosis of MS for more than twenty years before receiving a firm diagnosis this past year. She is self-employed as a special education consultant and dabbles in writing, art, and public speaking. Her condition is stable for now; she uses a walker, a power wheelchair, or whatever else is needed to allow her to perform her work duties.

We call her "Boss Lady" because of the advances we've witnessed in her professional life. She dreams of owning a spiritual arts center where she and her son (who has mild autism) "can find useful and fulfilling employment and touch the lives of others."

▲▲▲

BARB, forty, and her husband have four children, ages eleven to twenty-six. She's the material control manager for a large furniture manufacturer. In her spare time, she plays the violin, piano, and organ, plays with her cats, and reads. She was diagnosed in 1994, and her MS has been mild so far.

I'm very thankful for the insights I've received by having MS in my life, and very, very thankful for my online "Sisters."

▲▲▲

MARGE, at sixty-three, is the oldest member of the Froup, our "Exalted Crone." She had to retire in 1984 because of lifelong undiagnosed medical problems. MS was diagnosed in 1986 and fibromyalgia in 1997. She has had celiac disease (see the glossary) since early childhood. Her mobility symptoms have been relatively benign, but she has had major cognitive problems at times. She also has plaque in the autonomic areas of the brain, which causes blood pressure spikes, fluid retention, electrolyte imbalances, arrhythmia, and respiratory problems. Married, with adult children, she spends much of her time doing research on treating her combined ailments and on avoiding allergens and environmental factors that aggravate them.

My present joy in life comes from simple things, such as feeding birds, watching the deer, rabbits, squirrels, and chipmunks outside my back windows, planting things indoors and out, and reading messages from my "Sisters."

▲▲▲

KARON is married, with two stepchildren, and has been helping to raise her infant niece since the death of her sister-in-law in 1997. She was diagnosed in 1987 and is now in remission ("Shhh, don't jinx it!"). She worked as a school psychologist in Colorado, then as an accountant when she moved to Florida. She was training for a third career, as a paralegal, when the MS "started kicking the stuffing out of me." She enjoys spending her time quietly.

> *I don't talk much. Almost all my activities are things that I can do alone (reading, working puzzles, music, swimming, travel). Being in the Froup makes me feel good, not so lonely.*

Karon's contributions to our group discussions have become more numerous lately; we'll probably have to revise our assessment of her as the "quiet one" very soon.

▲▲▲

JOY, married to Jack and the mother of an adult daughter, Jen, is fifty-seven. She was in her late forties when diagnosed, after twenty years of worsening symptoms. She recently had to give up her job as an advertising writer (she has major problems with vertigo and fatigue) but is still able to do some freelance work. We call her "Saint Joy" because she always manages to come up with the "right" answer to any question on morals or ethics. She enjoys "genealogy, gemstones, gardening, and my countless nieces and nephews."

▲▲▲

SALLY, forty-seven, uses a wheelchair most of the time but still manages to live alone in a beachside apartment. Because of this, her nickname is "da Beachgirl." She trained her dog, Sandy, to be her helper/companion; she also has a pet snake. Sally's refrigerator (see Chapter Four) is the theoretical hiding place of many MSers' lost belongings.

▲▲▲

VICKI, forty, is married to Larry. They have young twins, Ash and Zach (it looks like Vicki tried to complete her family, from A to Z, in one fell swoop!). She uses a cane on short jaunts, a wheelchair or scooter on longer ones. She says that she's had to adapt to a license plate with a picture of a wheelchair; sitting to shower, cook, or wash dishes; fat pens that won't fly out of her hands; sticking a needle in her leg every week; and taking antidepressants. "But every day that I wake up *above* ground is a good day!"

▲▲▲

DONNA is forty-one, married, and has three children. Her special joy in life is the time spent with her four grandchildren. She was officially diagnosed in January of 1997. Shortly afterward, her symptoms forced her to retire from her job in the police department. Her nickname is "3-D Donna," mostly because her hands stutter when she tries to sign off ("D-D-Donna"). Lately, she has adopted another nickname, "Thray Day." She uses this when she writes to tell us about her fictional escapades through the Deep South. She's also our official biscotti baker (although we've yet to taste any of her creations. Hint, hint, Donna/3-D/Thray Day!).

▲▲▲

LYNN: That's me! I'm forty-nine; I've been married to Ron for the past twenty-eight years, and I have two daughters, Karen, twenty-seven, and Julie, twenty-five. I was diagnosed with "probable" MS in 1976; the diagnosis was confirmed in 1993 with an MRI. I had only occasional flare-ups, with full remissions in between, until 1990, when my symptoms became more progressive. I use canes, crutches, a wheelchair, a scooter, or whatever else is needed to maintain my "partially ambulatory" status. My biggest concern is my worsening cognitive problems; I consider it a true miracle that

I've been able to put this book together. I'd thought that my writing days were over when I had to retire from my job as an editorial assistant/reporter in 1991. My friends in the Froup call me "Lady Lynn." "Lynn" because that's my real middle name and the name I use online. The "Lady" part is a mystery.

3

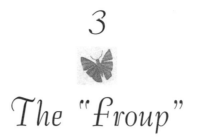

The "Froup"

JOY — This afternoon, I received a surprise phone call from an old buddy from Air Force days. Marilyn was the first person I ever knew well who had MS. I remember the day she first told me about it, back in 1976. It turned out that she'd already had her diagnosis for several years, but she seldom talked about it. She still doesn't talk about it much. But today she wanted to talk about MS. She needed to talk about it. And, as all of us have discovered, it is *so* much easier to discuss MS with another MSer.

Marilyn told me, "I seldom mention it to anyone else, because as soon as you say you have MS, people expect you to be in a wheelchair or something, and they look at you kinda funny, and I just don't want to deal with all that, and I don't want to be fussed over." Does that sound familiar?

She's using a cane now because her left leg has gotten so weak that she started falling a lot. She just finished a course of oral steroids . . . complete with bloating. Her vision is screwed up. When she looks at an "S," it's divided, like a dollar sign. She was the first to tell me, years ago, about some of the weird experiences that come with this disease. Back then, I didn't have any idea of what I was in for.

As we talked, though, I realized how much of what she was saying is now very familiar to me. Not because I've gone through all of it myself, but because at least one person in our group has gone through just about any weird thing the rest of us could think up. It reminded me again of how much our Froup means to me. I wish Marilyn (who isn't online) had Sisters like y'all to chat with on a regular basis so she wouldn't feel so alone with the disease. I wish we could share what we have here with the whole world of MSers. I guess the point of all this to say that we are a very fortunate bunch, because we have one another. The world could use a good dose of the love and caring we share in our Sisterhood. Wouldn't it be a nicer place to live and raise your family?

▲▲▲

For people with MS, the pursuit of such simple things as information, support, and socialization can be a daily challenge. Many of us aren't able to get out of the house much to scour libraries or bookstores for medical or other news. We don't have the stamina, endurance, or opportunity to pursue an active social life, search out new friends, and form strong relationships. If we use canes or wheelchairs or have other obvious differences, we may be uncomfortable in new situations with "normal" people. Our cognitive difficulties tend to flare up when we're in unfamiliar environments, in encounters with anyone but our closest friends and family members, so we avoid situations where this might occur.

Once in a while, though, we need to "leave" our everyday surroundings and seek out a safe place where we can talk about our ups and downs with others who are going or have gone through the same experiences.

I discovered a place like that one day in late 1996 when I was browsing through a medical area on the Internet. I found an assembly of more then twenty bulletin boards, each dealing with a different aspect of life with MS. Here, people who deal with multiple sclerosis, as patients or as family members or as caregivers, ask and answer questions about their own experiences and those of others who post to the boards.

At first, I was a bit hesitant to get involved in the on-screen discussions. I'd gone to support group meetings when I was first diagnosed with MS, more than twenty years ago. While sometimes good information was disclosed by doctors and patients at these meetings, there wasn't any true sharing with one another. There was no emotional involvement, no real feeling for one another. I think we were all hesitant to expose ourselves and become vulnerable to the other members of the group. Those of us who were still ambulatory, without need for any kind of assistive devices, told ourselves that we'd never get as bad as those around us in wheelchairs or on crutches. That's what I thought, anyway. We must have feared that the more experienced MSers there, those whose conditions had progressed to a more "disabled" level, would view us newbies as uninformed rookies who didn't know anything about life with something as daunting as MS. At the same time, it was hard to be confronted with the real possibility that we, too, might end up just as debilitated, using those same wheelchairs and crutches.

While the online message boards were less intimidating than in-person meetings, I still held back. I'd heard so many scary things about meeting people on the Internet. How seemingly innocent friendships turned into dangerous entanglements. How one little slip in safety or security measures could result in financial or emotional devastation. So I proceeded very cautiously. I introduced myself simply as "Lynn," my middle name. I read the posts till I got a feel for what was going on and for the level of sharing that took place. Then I answered a few of them, simple words of support or encouragement ("Oh, yes, I know what you mean," or "I hope you feel better soon"), but I offered little input about myself.

After a couple of weeks of this kind of lurking, though, I found myself getting to know the authors of the messages, to care about their triumphs and trials as they went about living with the Mon-Ster. I felt compelled to join in and share mine, too. Eventually I became friends with each of the ladies in our group.

We call ourselves the Sisterhood of Flutterbuds, since our founding members met and began corresponding on the "Mental Flutters" bulletin board. All of us are women. At various times, male MSers have expressed interest in participating in our exchange; there are men who contribute, in a very constructive way, to the bulletin boards, and we appreciate their input there. But to encourage the ease of conversation inherent to an all-one-sex membership, we've ended up with just women for our round-robin letters.

I'll let Helen tell you more about how our group came into being. She wrote this shortly after some of our members, though scattered to the four corners of the United States, pulled together to locate, finance, and deliver two air conditioners for another member who was going through an especially bad MS exacerbation during the summer heat. This was the point at which we realized that more good could come from our gathering than merely creating a place to gossip about an illness.

▲▲▲

HELEN — Some months ago, I started reading the "Mental Flutters" board and responding to some of the stuff people wrote there. A particular group of us got "into" this and started sharing things in our personal lives that made us laugh, or things that made us cry, or just things that we needed to tell someone. A few people got ticked because we were making this a "coffee klatch" instead of discussing our cognitive problems with MS. So, Renee tried to get us a subject board of our own, but that didn't work out. . . .

One morning I logged on [to the Internet] and there was what can only be described as a *shitload* of mail in my box! Someone (Renee?) had started a round-robin mailing, so that everyone could keep in touch without offending those who wanted to post strictly "by the boards." Day by day, as we all sent and received the letters, we learned one another's names, shared our sorrows and joys, began to tease one another.

Eventually we "shook down" to the cohesive group of cyber-friends that we now have become.

It was at this time that I began to seriously consider writing a book about life with the MonSter. I realized that anything presented from my point of view alone would not be at all comprehensive. I'd read several books by authors with MS and ended up feeling left out when I read accounts of symptoms or episodes that I'd never experienced. Likewise, I felt "overly endowed" when I read something from an MSer whose symptoms were milder than mine. This mystery disease varies too much from one person to the next to be described accurately through only one person's experiences.

Then I realized that right there on my computer screen was a gold mine of information about life with MS. It came straight from the hearts of, and was constantly replenished by, women who were examples of that life at each of its stages. I presented my idea to the Flutterbuds and was thrilled when they agreed to participate in the creation of this book.

The collection of these anecdotes has been an enlightening, humbling project for me. I'm amazed at the knowledge that these people have accumulated about MS and similar disorders. Compared to most of them, I was virtually ignorant. The whole medical-management side of multiple sclerosis has changed greatly since I was first diagnosed. Since then, I'd mostly concentrated on the personal survival side of it and neglected to keep a close eye on current findings in the field. Many of the other Flutterbuds had kept up, though; most of my recently updated education about MS and the treatments available for it has come from them or sources they've recommended.

I'm even more awed by the wisdom and courage with which my "MS sisters" face the challenges of living with recurring, eventually progressive, disability. My cyber-association with them has boosted me emotionally, spiritually, and sometimes, at least in an indirect way, physically. They're the first ones I go to for the encouragement, inspiration, and, more often than not, large doses of humor that I need to get through days when the MonSter is most bothersome. I consider each of them my friend, my comrade, my teacher, my sister.

Our purpose in this book isn't to distribute stark medical knowledge about multiple sclerosis. Very little of the medical information reported in these pages is quoted from documented findings of scientifically designed studies. It mostly comes from the very people who deal with multiple sclerosis daily, who are all personally familiar with the disease and what it can do to its prey. All the experiences are shared in a conversational context, and are not intended as medical advice.

Multiple sclerosis isn't our only, or even our primary, topic of conversation. The disease touches our lives in every area, it's true. But each of us has chosen to pursue, as actively as possible, a life independent of MS's influence. So we end up talking about children and grandchildren, marriages, careers, hobbies, music, movies, pets, and everything else that non-MSers talk about.

Sometimes we just have fun. We've assembled our own "Flutterbuds' dictionary" to keep track of new words we've invented to describe the quirky events in our lives. (Some examples—"Froup" is an abbreviation of "Flutterbuds' group." "Stribble" is what an MSer does when she attempts to remove her clothes fast enough to make it to the toilet before the dribbles start.) We fantasize, sometimes jokingly and sometimes seriously, about someday having joint ownership of a place called "Fogbound Ranch" where people with MS can go for rest, recreation, education, medical care, and anything else that we believe would improve our lives.

Helen and some of the other Flutterbuds share more about the unique bond that has formed among us.

▲▲▲

HELEN — Aside from the fact that we all have MS, an observer would think that we're all too different from one another to find anything in common to talk about. I guess that's true, to a certain extent. Some of us are married with kids; some are married without kids; some aren't married. We come from all walks of life and many socioeconomic levels. Our educations, lifestyles, sexual orientations, careers, ages, likes, and dislikes are all over the place, as are we. Yet, from the deep Ol' South to the far Northwest, we're all in the same place, no matter where we may physically live.

We've come to know one another's significant others, kids, parents, in-laws, outlaws, neighbors, friends, and pets. Yet not more than a half-dozen of us have met face-to-face. We grieve one another's losses, we have conniptions when one of us is sick, we laugh at ourselves and at one another. We are Catholic, Protestant, Jewish, Muslim, pagan, and unbeliever, and we never lose respect for one another's different points of view. We share recipes, pets, household hints, medical information, and lots of love baboons [one Flutterbud's typo when talking about the "love balloons" we send to cheer each other. This is one of the terms that made it into our Flutterbuds' Dictionary]. We offer each other online companionship during the long, dark nights when we can't sleep, either because we're sick or because we're scared. . . .

We're poets and artists and cooks and housewives and social workers and dreamers . . . and each one is as important as the next. We are a true democracy, in which everyone has an equal voice.

Nothing happens by coincidence. We came together for a reason. Our meeting was anything but happenstance. Five years down the road, who knows where we'll all be, if the Flutterbuds will have gone our separate ways, or if we'll still be together with yet another purpose? But here and now, there is a reason for us to just be.

The support level and the level of understanding in this group are simply astounding. I was in a "real" support group after I was first diagnosed, and I was bored silly. None of those people who met every week had a chance to know one another enough to really care about one another. The love and caring in this group never cease to astonish me.

We have varying levels of physical functioning. Of "fogginess." But, while each of us may not be able to do everything, together we can do *anything!* Finding air conditioners for our FlutterSis last summer is just a small example of what a bunch of determined women with "disabilities" can do. We may not always be able to tie our shoes, but we can work miracles.

I love all of you.

▲▲▲

DONNA — I think that our group connection is spiritual (which is different from religious) in the bond that has formed and the way our personalities blend and complement one another. Our multiple egos come together to make a separate being of power, love, and commitment. Sometimes I get so caught up in reading the mail that circulates here, watching the flow of love and acceptance, that I forget I am part of this big, wonderful being. I forget to respond as I marvel at the wisdom, kindness, and compassion moving back and forth between the Sisters. This gathering of warm, wonderful souls could not have been by accident.

▲▲▲

HELEN again — I grew up with a lot of Native American tradition. One thing many of the tribes teach is that we are all relatives. They refer to the world, visible and invisible, as "all my relations." When I live in a city, as I do now, I walk pretty much the same path that everyone else does. When I go out into the woods, which is my chapel/church/temple, I become someone else, so aware of what my "relatives" are doing. We are all connected in this wonderful circle, and we are all a part of everything. Some Indians refer to white people as "the people that make things square," in reference to houses, buildings, garden plots, etc., and say that this has caused us to lose the "circle" of interconnectedness.

I think that because our members are spread all over, rather than confined to one village, town, city, or whatever, we are regaining this circularity. That's why we're so attuned to one another in the Froup.

A group like ours, coming from all over the States, all with multiple sclerosis, all coping the way we do, with support from people we talk to online every day, could be inspirational to others who have this disease. [And maybe for those who don't have this disease as well!] We have all been made much stronger and learned many coping skills by communicating with one another. We have gained much inner strength, and it seems that whenever we need a "boost," the material for it is right there in our pool, waiting to be tapped.

The Internet and the online services get so much bad publicity. Our group could do a lot to promote the good side of online communication. We're not out to cause trouble or raise hell via the services; we're not info-junkies surfing the Net for sport. We're basically here just to communicate. And communicate we do!

My housemate said one day that while she doesn't believe in "fate" or "predestination" most of the time, this bunch was intended by The Powers That Be to meet. And we make the most of it, right?

▲▲▲

RENEE — Just gotta share this with y'all. The other day, I was at the school and heard something (can't remember what it was now) and remarked to the person speaking, "I'm going to tell my Sisters this one." This lady said, "Oh, I always wanted a sister. How many do you have?" And without a skip I said, "Oh, twenty-five or thirty; I can never remember exactly."

You should have seen the look on her face! I didn't realize what I'd said until after the conversation, when I was on the way back to my car.

JAMIE — In this group, we have a bond that is stronger than the chains and weights of this damned disease. Though we may not know all the faces, we do know all the hearts!

Maybe we can't walk, but together we fly!

4

If It Looks Like a Duck…

LORI — Today was my appointment with the only neurologist on the "Good Docs List" for our entire state. I failed my neurological exam! Hooray for me! He was not exactly pleased with the way I was treated by my last doctor, and he is planning more tests that were not run previously. They may lead to other tests, but we are just going to try one thing at a time so I don't have to go through the testing marathon again. And guess what? I am not crazy! I don't even have an anxiety disorder, which is what Dr. P. told me I had when I saw him right after I started having health problems. Oh, how I love this new guy. He actually spoke to me like a human being and as if I might have the slightest modicum of intelligence. *He even has a personality!*

Steve came with me to the doctor's today and got to see the things that turned out abnormally on the exams. My reflexes are not right, and I have rather severely diminished feeling in my fingers and toes. I wasn't even aware of this. I can feel when they go completely numb, when I feel like they belong to someone else, but I didn't know that there was an ongoing problem. That was a shocker for me. The doctor does seem to think the eye problems I've been having are due to ocular migraines and silent migraines; he will formulate a plan to get them under control. I told him about the big problem with light sensitivity and that I don't want to continue living like a vampire. He thought that was funny.

I told him that I am not necessarily looking for a firm diagnosis, but that I need a doctor who will stick with me and be supportive of whatever is going on and not write it off to anxiety. He told me I definitely have a whole lot more going on than anxiety. Well, duh! I wish he would call up that other doctor and yell at him. It was odd to leave the doctor's office happy that I had an abnormal neurological exam. Too funny. Steve was happy, too. Not happy that it was abnormal, of course, but we've just been going through this for so long that it felt really nice to be . . . damn, what's that word? I keep thinking *vindicated* or *justified*, but that's not it . . . *validated!* I hate word searching. What a strain it puts on the brain!

Ooooh, by the way, this doctor actually said that diagnostics (series of tests used to diagnosis an illness) are a weak tool and not always accurate, but that they're pretty much the only tools they have to go by, which makes diagnosis difficult! I can't believe he admitted that. I was shocked and thrilled all at the same time. He said that that doesn't mean I don't have something going on, because it's obvious by the neurological exam that I do. So, *ha!* Dr. P., stick that in your anxiety-disorder diagnosis!

▲▲▲

Is this possible? A young wife and mother suspects that she has a catastrophic medical problem, and she rejoices when a doctor tells her that she's probably right? If that young woman is experiencing the first signs and symptoms of multiple sclerosis, it's not only possible, it's very likely. Like Lori, many of us have concluded that anything is better than those typical first days or months or years with multiple sclerosis, when there are no answers to explain the strange happenings within our bodies.

Since it was first identified in the middle of the nineteenth century, multiple sclerosis has been considered a "mystery" disease. Diagnosis has at times been a maddeningly vague process, largely a guessing game. At best, it was a matter of ruling out other conditions when possible and then naming whatever was left "multiple sclerosis." Just a couple of decades ago, MS was usually the last tag pasted onto a set of symptoms. Even now, with so much more sophisticated diagnostic technology in use, the disorder can masquerade as many others, making for a long and winding road to a positive diagnosis.

Multiple sclerosis is usually diagnosed by a neurologist, a specialist in disorders of the nervous system. Prior to that, though, the patient typically has symptoms that aren't overtly neurological: maybe a bout with double vision, which sends the patient to an ophthalmologist; or bladder malfunctions, which send the patient to a urologist; or a collection of "vague" complaints, maybe accompanied by depression, that seem to call for psychiatric care. Many times the doctor, whatever his or her specialty, suspects MS and refers the person to a neurologist.

That's when the fun begins. The first step is an examination, along with a detailed medical history tracing the symptoms that precipitated the visit. Often other diseases, some of which may be similar to MS in their initial appearance (myasthenia gravis and Lyme disease, among others) can be ruled out at this time. If he or she feels it's necessary, the doctor may then order a spinal tap, which detects abnormalities in the spinal fluid, or evoked response tests, which measure the length of time it takes for outside stimuli to reach the brain. One of the most conclusive tests used now is magnetic resonance imaging, or MRI, which can show telltale spots (MS lesions) on the brain and spinal cord.

No one of these tests is infallible in coming up with a diagnosis. It may be necessary to perform all of them, and yet others, before a physician can make a definite judgment. Usually, too, since the disease by definition involves multiple trouble spots in the nervous system, the doctor waits for more than one symptom to show up before making a final pronouncement.

In rare cases, the patient breezes through the diagnostic process with a doctor who discovers exactly the right set of signs and symptoms at the very first visit or performs a certain test at exactly the right moment. I actually met one of these singular souls; I shared a room with her in the outpatient department of the hospital where we'd both gone for treatment of MS flare-ups. This lady, a registered nurse, had had several visual and sensory problems that she recognized as possibly neurological in origin. So she went to a neurologist, who examined her, took her history, and sent her for an MRI. Twenty minutes after the test was completed, the neurologist (who, by the way, is the one that I see now) was able to say, "You have multiple sclerosis."

Most of us have to go through a much longer process to come up with something conclusive. My own diagnostic experience would probably be rated as average in its duration and intensity.

In the winter of 1970–71, Ron and I were busy celebrating an assortment of momentous firsts: our first wedding anniversary, the purchase of our first home, and the anticipated arrival of our first child. I was in my sixth month of pregnancy, just beginning to look and feel somewhat ungainly and awkward. I was uncomfortable with, but very proud of, my ever-increasing girth. The baby was obviously growing well and was already enjoying a very active lifestyle. It had evolved, in the depths of my consciousness, from a lump in my lower belly to a living, loved presence in my life. I'd gotten over my morning sickness, given up my job, and granted free rein to my nesting instincts, which coaxed me into sleeping late in the mornings and sewing curtains for the nursery in the afternoons. I was content, and I couldn't envision myself or anyone else in my household being anything other than content for as long as we lived. I was complacently unaware that another first was in our immediate future: I was about to have my first encounter with the disease that would become one of the most encompassing, demanding, commanding, compelling, directing forces in my family's life.

In spite of my contentment, that winter seemed to drag on. There was so much to look forward to, and I was impatient with waiting. Then February brought one more reason for me to wish that spring would come and, with it, the delivery of my baby. I began to experience weird sensations in my legs, a protest, I assumed, against the extra burden they were forced to carry. Often when I changed positions suddenly, especially when I stood up, the normal, benign, unnoticeable feeling in my legs disappeared. It was replaced by a wild tingling sensation, exactly how I imagined it would feel to stand on an electrically charged floor mat. Concurrent surges of searing heat and icy cold rushed from my toes to my groin. All the nerves in the lower half of my body seemed to crackle; I almost expected to self-incinerate at any second. I was effectively paralyzed; if I dared to move another muscle once this began, the sensation spread up my spine and down my arms, all the way to my fingertips. (I later learned that this was an exaggerated manifestation of Lhermitte's sign, an electrical tingling along the spine which is common in many disorders involving the spinal cord. Even by itself, it can be a valuable clue in diagnosing MS.) I tried to remain perfectly still for as long as the prickling, stinging, zinging continued, anywhere from a few seconds to several minutes. After it subsided, I was left absolutely zapped, as though I'd experienced an actual electric shock. My extremities were numb, heavy, clumsy at best and immobile at worst. That part of it, the deadness, continued for as long as several days at a time. Gradually, the feeling and the vitality returned, and I could go back to concentrating on getting ready for my baby.

I was concerned that I'd fall and hurt the baby during one of those "attacks." Other than that, there didn't seem to be much reason for alarm. I just put the blame on my inability to adjust quickly enough to my own ungainliness. My obstetrician, when I mentioned the problem to him, agreed. He assured me that the baby was most likely sitting on a nerve, and that the "electric episodes" would disappear once I delivered.

The shocks, however, continued to plague me for months after Karen's birth in May of 1971. I still didn't worry much. With a bright, vivacious baby in the house, there was too much else to think about and to expend time and energy on. Besides, the attacks were mild and short-lived compared to those I'd had during pregnancy. When I thought about it at all, I assumed that whatever nerve had been "sat on" was still in the process of healing.

That blissful unawareness saw me through the next few years. Looking back now, I know that certain events during that time should have warned me that something was still wrong. I'd lost the vision in my left eye for several weeks (the doctor called it iritis). I'd had days-long episodes of a kind of mildly dizzy disorientation, accompanied by alternating bouts of constipation and diarrhea (attributed to a spastic colon). I'd gone through periods of crushing, debilitating depression for which I couldn't find any logical reason. My internist, Dr. S., finally referred me to Dr. A. for psychotherapy, hoping to alleviate all my strange symptoms in the process. Dr. A. treated me for extended postpartum blues, and life went on.

It didn't occur to me to try to string all these things together as part of anything apart from the depression. I was too busy to dwell on my problems: Julie was born in 1973, when Karen was two years old, and Ron's job took him out of town several days a week. That left me with limited time to correlate a lot of seemingly unrelated little medical annoyances. Besides, it wasn't as if I found a new problem every day or had any of the old ones for more than a few days at a time. The one problem that remained constant was the depression; that became my catch-all explanation for the assortment of small, come-and-go annoyances that plagued me.

Then, on an afternoon in mid-October, 1975, everything changed. Ron was working second shift, and I'd been trying to do some fall cleanup in the yard. For most of the day, I'd felt "funny," in a way that I couldn't describe even to myself. Late in the afternoon, my mother stopped in for a visit. I was glad for the company and asked Mom to stay for supper, which was to be a bucket of chicken from the Colonel. She offered to watch the kids while I went out to pick up the food.

At the first stop sign, I realized that my brakes didn't work correctly. I thought I was pushing the pedal to the floor, but the car didn't stop. I drove slowly back to the house, where Mom told me to leave my car and take hers. At the same stop sign, I discovered that her brakes didn't work, either. Back at the house, Mom just looked at me kind of funny when I reported the problem to her. She went out and tried the brakes; they worked perfectly for her. So we put the girls in the car, and Mom drove us all to get the chicken.

Sometime that evening, I became aware that I couldn't feel my feet. It wasn't the tingling-followed-by-deadness sensation I'd had years earlier. It was just a pure absence of feeling. I didn't make much of it, except to remark to Mom that we didn't have to worry about getting the brakes checked on the cars; we just had to worry about getting my head checked again. I was sure that I was imagining the whole thing.

When Ron came home from work later that night, he took the situation more seriously and spent a long time trying to massage the sensation back into my feet. By the next day, though, the lack of feeling had crept up my legs. I'd recently stopped taking all my medications for depression, and I wondered if I was having some kind of withdrawal symptoms. When I checked with Dr. A., my psychiatrist, he said it was possibly a kind of anxiety reaction. That seemed logical; it was, in fact, what I'd expected to hear. I knew that I sometimes reacted strangely and strongly to anxieties that I wasn't even aware of. My regular session with Dr. A. was already scheduled for two weeks later, so we agreed to wait until then before deciding on a treatment.

In the meantime, the loss of sensation advanced all the way up to my waist. I was still too ignorant or naive to be concerned. The numbness seemed to be only skin deep; I could still function almost normally, as long as I literally watched my step.

Within a couple of days, though, it became obvious that the anesthesia went deeper than the skin. All of a sudden, I could no longer feel my bladder, so I had no idea of when it was filled beyond capacity. A couple of times, before I figured out what was going on, it overflowed on its own without any warning. I caught on very quickly that it was going to be up to me to empty it often enough to prevent that from happening again. But it was useless to attempt to go before sufficient pressure had built up. My bladder refused to pay attention to my brain's message that it was okay to go *now*. At that time, Julie was two years old and recently potty-trained. I ended up borrowing her leftover disposable diapers every time I had to leave the house during the two weeks before my appointment.

Somewhere in those weeks, I talked to Mom. "I can't even feel when I have to pee," I laughed.

She didn't laugh. All she said was, "Oh, honey!" Then she paused and said again, "Oh, honey!"

The fear in her voice sent a jolt of awareness through me. There was *something wrong*. For the first time, I was really scared.

Somehow I made it through those weeks. I adopted a kind of spraddled, stiff-legged waddle to propel myself around enough to take care of my kids. On the day of my appointment, my sister Sandy offered to drive me. She came directly from a dental visit to pick me up, with both sides of her face still paralyzed from Novocain. On the way to Dr. A.'s office, we joked about the possibility of getting a group rate for treatment when he saw the two of us.

Dr. A. didn't seem to think there was anything to joke about. "You should have called me back when it got worse," he said. He picked up the phone right away and made arrangements for me to see a neurologist, Dr. M., the next morning at the hospital emergency room.

Ron and I went to the appointment unprepared to spend any time in the hospital beyond the hour or so needed for the examination. Without even having to convince myself, I was sure that Dr. M. would send me right back to Dr. A. with a diagnosis of hypochondria.

At first, Dr. M. seemed to concur with my judgment—he made several offhand allusions to the fact that I'd been referred by a psychiatrist, saying that I shouldn't expect him to find an instant physical explanation for my symptoms. After his exam, though, he sent Ron to pick up the personal items I'd need during some time away from home, and to arrange care for Karen and Julie. In the meantime, he admitted me to the hospital and started a series of diagnostic procedures. The next few days were a jumble of bright lights, whirring motors, needle punctures, knee taps, constant discomfort, and a million questions asked of me and by me.

But no answers, at least not to my questions. Dr. M. came in after each day of testing and reported on the disorders he'd been able to rule out that day. By the end of the fourth day, I knew I didn't have a brain or spinal tumor, myasthenia gravis, spinal cord injury, or a number of other conditions. On the fifth day, Dr. M. performed a spinal tap. Later that day, the atmosphere in my room seemed to somehow change. Until then, when I needed something, I had to push the call button and wait for a nurse to answer. Now a nurse seemed to be hovering nearby at all times, ready to instantly tend to my needs. The staff social worker showed up with information about resources that would be available if I needed help to care for my family. It was pretty obvious that some new bit of information had been posted to my medical chart, that all the test results had at last added up to something positive.

It was also obvious that the something positive was serious. Why else would this young lady be seated at my bedside, reviewing lists of agencies that I could call for help with child care? Half of my mind wanted to whisper calm thanks for her concern. The other half was screaming, "Why are you telling me these things? What is it that you're *not* telling me?" I couldn't manage to push the words from either half of my mind to my lips. I sat mutely while the social worker went through her spiel. Then, amazingly, I allowed her to get up and walk out of my room without answering any of my unasked questions.

By the next morning, I was fully convinced that I was dying. I hadn't slept at all. I had a grinding headache, a legacy of the spinal tap. I was exhausted, scared, and just plain sick of waiting for explanations. I missed my kids. I wanted to go home. I wanted to forget I'd ever thought about trying to find out what was wrong with me. By the time the breakfast trays were delivered, I'd worked myself into a state of total despair. I started to cry, and I couldn't stop.

Sometime that morning, Dr. A. showed up at my bedside. For about fifteen minutes, he didn't say anything. He just sat on the edge of the bed, held my hand, and let me cry. I knew that he knew what was wrong with me. Dr. M. had obviously conferred with him. I also knew that he wouldn't step into Dr. M.'s realm to tell me what it was.

Oddly enough, I felt a stirring of hope at that moment. If Dr. A. knew the diagnosis, then at least there was, finally, a diagnosis to know. And if my psychiatrist intended to leave it to my neurologist to give me the news, then it must be a real illness, something physical that could be dealt with, not just something I'd conjured in my twisted imagination.

Finally, as Dr. A. stood to leave, he spoke. "Will Ron be here this afternoon?" When I nodded, he said, "Okay, I'll let Dr. M. know."

Dr. M. came in during afternoon visiting hours, shortly after Ron's arrival. He again went through the list of illnesses that he'd ruled out. At the end, he said, ". . . so my conclusion is that you probably have multiple sclerosis."

I had no idea what that meant. But as Dr. M. went on to say that he would begin immediately to treat it with injections of ACTH, that I would go through physical therapy to help me regain full use of my legs, and that I'd have to spend a couple more weeks in the hospital, I didn't really care what it meant. I just grabbed onto the realization that I had something that could be treated, that there was hope that I'd walk on my own again, and that I'd be able to leave the hospital before the end of the world.

The only questions in my mind hinged on his use of the word

probably. I wanted assurance that this was finally the end of wondering. I wanted some certainty that I could just get on with my life. I simply asked, "Are you sure it's multiple sclerosis?"

He answered, "With MS, we can't be absolutely sure, at least not until the patient dies and we can do an autopsy and look at the brain and spinal cord." (This was in the pre-MRI era.) He headed off my next question ("Am I going to die?") with "Don't worry, you've got quite a few years to go yet before we'll do that."

That was enough information for me. I finally had a name for the MonSter that had been stalking me, and the assurance that I had some time to come to terms with its presence in my life. I was too tired, and in some ways too relieved, to ask for more.

I lived with the "probable MS" verdict for the next fifteen years. At that point, my newest neurologist (by that time, I'd seen three), Dr. R., ordered an MRI. An hour later, he pointed out to me the clusters of white spots on the image of my brain, leaving no doubt about the diagnosis.

I guess there's no "best" way to find out that you have a chronic, progressive disease. But, looking back on it, especially after hearing the stories of others who have gone through diagnosis, I'm grateful that my experience took the course it did. There wasn't the trauma of a sudden, shocking revelation; nor did I have to endure an interminable period of wondering. While four years elapsed between the time my first symptoms showed up and the time of the "probable" diagnosis, they weren't four years of conscious concern about what was wrong with me. It was more like four years of getting used to the idea, just barely formed on the fringes of my awareness, that my myriad little problems would someday be lumped together under the name of one big, bad disease.

▲▲▲

BREN — One fall day (I don't remember the month), I "cracked" my neck . . . you know, like cracking knuckles. Well,

I went numb and tingly from the neck down. I thought, "Oh, *great!* I just paralyzed myself!" Anyway, I had to see my doctor that day for a cold, so I told him about it. He gave me some ibuprofen, which seemed to ease the bit of swelling in my neck that we felt was arthritis. Eventually, *most* of the numbness went away, but my hands and feet were still numb. I was losing strength in both as well. I went back to the doctor, and he immediately made an appointment with the local neurologist, saying, "That's not normal, and I don't want to mess around with it."

So I headed to the neurologist. He did a thorough exam, including the evoked potential tests. (I think that's what they're called . . . where they stick the little electrodes on your skull, and have you sit there, watching patterns on a computer screen. Then you lie in a chair with the same electrodes on, and listen to very quiet sounds, beeps, etc. I fell asleep in that one.) Anyway, he looked at those results and did reflex tests, minor ones with the little hammer, and had me walk across the room a few times. Then he turned to me and said, "I suspect MS, multiple sclerosis, but I can't be sure."

As with many of us, I knew *nothing* about the nature of the Beast. So I asked him, "What do you mean, you suspect? Aren't there any more tests you can run?"

He said "Yes, I'll have you get an MRI." So I went off and got the MRI. I had a second appointment with him about two weeks later, after he got the results. We sat there in his office, and he said again, "I suspect MS, but I can't be sure." I was thinking, *say what?* So I asked again. "Isn't there some other test you can do to make sure?"

He said we *could* do a spinal tap; *however*, he was *very* uncomfortable doing a tap on me. He did not want to do *any* invasive procedures at all! So I went home.

For the next three years, I did my own thing, just boppin' along. I had myself convinced that it *was* really arthritis, and that this neurologist was nuts. For those three years, I just hung in there.

Then, one evening during dance rehearsals for *West Side Story* (I was one of the girls in the chorus), my feet started feeling tingly. I kind of dismissed it because we'd been stomping around a lot that night. We were close to performance dates, and so we'd started dancin' just for the fun of it.

Anyway, that evening I got home and lay down on my couch. My feet had what I now refer to as a "zinging" or "buzzing" sensation, like bees under the skin, this really weird thing going on, and I felt antsy all over. Then, about three hours later, my hands and feet went numb again, and it [numbness] was traveling up my arms and legs.

So I figured maybe I should check with a neurologist, but I didn't want to go back to that "idiot" (the one who said I might have MS). So I called around to pediatric neurologists (I got the list of referrals from my kids' doctor, and failed to mention that it was for *me!*), and who does *each and every one of them* recommend? You guessed it . . . that "idiot"! So I took their word for it and headed back to him. He recognized me immediately, which totally shocked me but also pleased me. He ordered another MRI, and when he got the results in a few days, I had another office visit.

Doc: "Okay, *now* I can tell you that you have multiple sclerosis."

Me: "Wait a minute . . . why couldn't you tell me that three years ago?"

Doc: "One word: Multiple. Three years ago, that didn't apply to you, because you only had problems stemming from one area of your central nervous system."

One word, ladies. *Duh!* Multiple! So we discussed options for treatment, etc. He told me that my prognosis was *fabulous*, and he'd be surprised if I ever had to use a cane or any walking aids. He said I had an extremely mild case of relapsing/remitting MS (and he explained it to me completely). He answered all my stupid questions and asked about memory loss, fatigue, headaches, urination, etc. I left the office with a prescription for an NSAID (nonsteroidal anti-inflammatory drug) for the migraines I'd been getting, and that was it. But I felt so very comfortable talking with him, and *knew* I could call him for any reason. He'd told me as much. Even if I just felt down or wanted to ask some questions or just needed to touch base with him to "feel better," he told me to call, day or night.

So, that's my diagnosis story. Not too awfully exciting, and not too bad as far as tests, etc. Thinking back now, I'm *glad* he didn't decide to "test me to death"!

▲▲▲

TARA — I first noticed that something was wrong when I was pregnant with my second son. I was twenty at the time. I had dizzy spells, and some days I had vertigo all the time. When I was pregnant with my third son, I was all of twenty-one, and the doctor had me go for a CAT scan because of the same symptoms. He saw nothing on the scan but noted that one pupil was smaller than the other and was fixed.

This all stayed about the same until my youngest was three. That's when I started having numbness in my hands and what felt like ants crawling in them. My doctor ran tests and found carpal tunnel syndrome. He did bilateral surgery, and I was better for a while; then the symptoms returned.

As the years went by, my doctor sent me off to various neurologists and rheumatologists because I was having joint pain and was pulling neck and arm muscles, and I had what appeared to be a TIA (a ministroke) that was right-sided and resulted in a bit of a droopy eyelid. They saw "soft" signs, but nothing they could put a finger on. My MRIs were fine. I had developed a slipped disc in my lower back by the time my youngest was five, and I ended up in traction until the orthopedic surgeon said that the disc could not be causing all the trouble. I had trouble walking; my feet felt like lead and I couldn't lift them. Still the MRIs were normal. The neurologist saw that I had position loss in my left big toe. He was startled by this and mentioned MS for the first time. Then my primary-care doctor noted my hyper reflexes and said, almost under his breath, "You know, you may really have MS."

Some time later, I was walking in a grocery store and my vision disappeared totally, instantly, for about twenty minutes. I was sent off to the emergency room, where they could find nothing wrong. From this point on, I had double vision, cloudy vision, etc., coming on and then fading out. I started to get that thing where electricity goes running down the spine when you move your head, and I got to where my upper back and arms were really weak.

I was tested for lupus, Lyme disease, myasthenia gravis, thyroid problems, and arthritis, over and over and over. Nothing ever showed up. Different doctors said I had very different things, like chemical diabetes, arthritis, Reynaud's syndrome, and fibromyalgia. And then they started telling me that maybe my doctor should have me see a psychiatrist. After fifteen years of this, I was having major trouble with fatigue and trouble walking; my legs would just buckle. I had incredible pain. I constantly pulled and strained my neck and upper back muscles. Every time this happened, I was sent for tests and they'd say, "Strained muscles, nothing else."

In 1991, I left my husband and moved away with the kids. The stress of that situation kicked up all my symptoms. I was also an emotional basket case, as I had just gotten out of a fifteen-year marriage to a highly controlling, emotionally and sexually abusive partner. I was diagnosed with manic/depressive disorder, which was later deleted from all my records and listed as post-traumatic shock.

My ex harped at me constantly that I should exercise and

that I would feel better if I got in shape. My family—parents, sister, brother—didn't have a clue about what was happening. They thought I was mentally unbalanced, because if there was something wrong, the doctors would have found it. They thought that they were doing me a big favor by "letting" me make my own way through all this. I ended up living in a place that I would not put a dog in.

I began to get weaker, and my legs got more and more involved. I had internal and then external tremors. I would fall asleep in my car at noon in order to get through the day at work. I had had enough at that point, and I told my mom that I had to have help or I was just going to die someday and they were all going to say, "Hey, what happened to her? I thought it was all in her head." So she went with me to the doctor. He listened to her, and we started the testing again. He did tons of tests and found nothing specific out of the ordinary (except the way the patient looked at that point). He did note, though, that there was absolutely something very wrong, and that he believed it to be MS.

At that point we stopped testing, since all the tests so far hadn't come up with anything, and I had no more patience and money to waste on tests that weren't helpful anyway. Then my primary-care physician (PCP) sent me again to the same neurologist, who still had no answers. He said that he would lean toward calling it lupus, and asked my PCP to test for that and some other things. He also said it could be MS, or maybe a cancer that was killing me and no one had found yet! My PCP knew that he had just done scans on my heart and my whole abdomen and had run every blood test in the world three times.

Finally he said, "Okay, we have ruled out this and this and this, and now we are left with MS. That's it." To this day, we do not have a positive MRI or spinal tap or any other positive test result. We have documented signs of two lesions (in the central nervous system). We could have documented more, but that was finally enough to say that my problem had to be MS.

I had gone to lots and lots of doctors, constantly, for twenty-two years. There were times I would stop for a couple of years because I didn't think I could bear any more. Then I would break down, find a new doctor, and try again. There were times (many, many) that I cried myself to sleep and just prayed that "someday" they would find out what was wrong.

As the MS progresses now, it is easier for me, because people see it, people can call it something, people want to help. Now it is accepted, and I don't have to cry myself to sleep over something harsh that someone said to me. I keep on going, keep working, keep striving and struggling, simply because there is no other choice.

I have learned so much in each situation that I had to live through and to conquer. I would never want to do it again, but the lessons learned are wonderful and have made me who I am today. I kind of like that person, so I guess it's all worth it.

▲▲▲

MARGE — You all know I'm the multidiseased Marge. I have had periods of illness all my life, since I was old enough to start being fed bread, crackers, cookies, etc. My MS symptoms showed up in my early teens, but most of them went untreated. Nothing ever was really resolved.

I married and had two children. My husband was killed during my pregnancy with my second child. When, with two toddlers, I decided to finish my education, I no longer had time to try to find out what was wrong.

When I'd get to the point where I'd come home so fatigued I could not even make it to the couch to lie down, I'd go to a doctor. Usually I'd get an antibiotic or something, and the problem would go away. Each time it happened, it took longer to recover. I started having clumsiness, increased "electrical jolts," muscle spasms, trouble remembering words I wanted, and increased pain in my bones, joints, and muscles, and the fatigue started to really bother me. I had difficulty sleeping even though I was exhausted.

By that time, I was forty-six years old and had remarried. I had periodic exacerbations of pain, spasm, fatigue, memory loss, etc., to the point where I'd work Monday and Tuesday, stay home Wednesday to get the pain under control, and then work Thursday and Friday.

By 1984, I had increased walking problems, mental problems, and pain. I would walk down a wide hall and go from one side to the other. I had serious shakiness. I was diagnosed with bipolar disorder. My primary-care doctor located the most highly respected psychiatrist in our area. I told him how worthless, frightened, paranoid, and claustrophobic I had become. He called in a wonderful clinical psychologist, who did some tests. They found that I had dropped twenty-five I.Q. points, lost organizational ability, and had severe short-term memory problems as well as coordination problems and noticeable changes in reaction rate.

At that time, my fighting spirit returned. I started spending my time in the medical library. In a month's time, I discovered the MS symptoms and found many similarities to what I was going through. I saw a neurologist, who said that there were only mild physical problems and that the cognitive problems didn't fit with MS. Nor did the pain.

A year later, in 1986, my alma mater was involved in developing the MRI. I was sent there for one. A few days later, my doctor called to tell me there were many plaques in the right frontal area of the brain. The university doctor was certain it was MS. I had a diagnosis. Although my MS symptoms had shown up in my early teens, nothing more was diagnosed until I was fifty-two years old.

I am optimistic, and certain that things can only improve.

As the problems that can be fixed are resolved, there will be less chance of triggering an MS exacerbation.

All of the people who thought it was "all in my head" were at least partially correct. It's in my head; it's also just about everywhere else in my body. . . .

▲▲▲

These five stories show the diversity in the diagnostic experience among MSers. I think that if I'd collected and included stories from all of our members, we'd now have twenty different tales. Each would tell of different first signs that hinted at serious illness; each would differ in the length of time from onset of symptoms to diagnosis; each would involve a different battery of tests, a different number of doctors' opinions. Even with today's improved diagnostic techniques, the process can be agonizingly slow.

Now, though, there are new reasons to forge ahead as quickly as possible in the search for a definitive diagnosis when MS is suspected. Recent research has proven that initiation of treatment with one of the new injectible drugs (copolymers and interferons) immediately after diagnosis can make a significant difference in the course of the disease. A swift diagnosis is necessary because virtually all insurance companies require a positive diagnosis before they'll pay for the treatment, which costs about $1,000 a month. Few people are able to afford the drug during the uninsured "possible MS" period.

With that in mind, I'd advise anybody facing a potential MS diagnosis to go for it! Immediately! Allow the hope of effective treatment to override the fear of an unfavorable finding. Ask your doctor for a referral to a neurologist who specializes in treating multiple sclerosis. Allow yourself to be "tested to death." If one symptom is present that seems to be MS-related, retrace the past ten or fifteen or twenty years and record any other signs or symptoms that could, even in some far-fetched way, also be connected with MS. Then tell your doctor about them.

still wonder how much faster and easier my own diagnostic experience might have been if I'd known enough to say to my first neurologist, "Right now my legs are numb and I can't control my bladder. A couple of years ago, I lost the vision in my left eye. I've been depressed off and on, for no obvious reason, for the past four years. I've had an electric sensation down my spine and through my arms and legs; this started four years ago when I was pregnant, and I still have it once in a while." I think my childhood convent training wouldn't allow me to say these things or to ask questions. In school, our superiors told us everything we were supposed to know, and we weren't to question anything. I had the idea that this attitude carried over to anybody in "authority," that a doctor would tell me what he wanted to tell me, and the rest was none of my business. Apparently he had the same idea.

Don't wait for your doctor to ask about any of your symptoms. My first neurologist didn't. Be your own patient advocate if necessary. Learn as much as you can about your symptoms and what might be behind them. Bug your doctor to dig further if you're not satisfied that he/she hasn't found anything. Don't settle for the passive and submissive attitude that I had: I didn't realize that I was allowed to tell my doctor what I was experiencing. I didn't have to wait for him to tell me what I should be experiencing, and I didn't have to accept it when he did. Ask questions.

No matter how quickly or how slowly your diagnosis arrives, keep in mind throughout the process that whatever you learn will more than likely be easier to deal with than having a lot of strange symptoms that nobody can explain. If you don't have multiple sclerosis, congratulations! and God bless you as you learn to overcome whatever is ailing you. If you do have multiple sclerosis, welcome to the club, and God bless you again! Your diagnosis will bring with it relief and grief. But it's not a reason to stop living.

Joy speaks for all of us about the fight to find a diagnosis and the mixed emotions that we experience when it's found:

▲▲▲

An Uncivil War

Trigger-happy troops, the renegade cells
breach the blood-brain barrier and attack
their own command center.
What's wrong with me?
Am I imagining things?
Crazed cannibals, they chew the fatty armor
protecting nerves and, like rats gnawing
on electrical cords, shred the sheaves and damage
the delicate, dangerous wires beneath.
Why am I so weak?
What is this tingling?
The currents short out. A light flickers.
An impulse falters. A circuit overloads.
Soundless pops, zips, flashes roam like silent
lightning through the complex system.
I can't see. . . . My legs are numb. . . . I'm so
dizzy. . . . I can't walk. . . . I'm very tired. . . . I can't
think straight. . . . I'm so clumsy. . . . The pain is back. . . .
I can't control. . . .
Guerrilla fighters, the killers strike at random,
retreat, regroup, and return in the night,
seeking to destroy, firing at anything that moves,
torching their own homes. . . .
unknowing, uncaring, unpredictable.
At least I have a diagnosis now.
I can name the enemy, and it will not defeat me.
Attitude is everything, and I will not surrender.
I'll get better soon. I know I will.
Scarred but serene, we sleep like battle-weary
soldiers, comforting each other, hoping to heal,
waiting for the next onslaught,
praying it never comes.
We have multiple sclerosis. Cause unknown.

5

Sally's Fridge and Other Flutters

One busy afternoon not long ago, I foraged through my freezer, looking for something that could be popped in the microwave for a quick supper. I found a storage container that looked interesting; perhaps it was the leftovers of a not-too-far-in-the-past meal that was good enough to be saved for a second go-round.

I looked at the label I'd attached to the top. "Rustproofing Sauce." In my handwriting. Rustproofing sauce? I couldn't remember the last time I'd used, or even heard of, anything vaguely resembling rustproofing sauce. And why would I have stored something like that in the freezer? Maybe Ron had brought it in from his workshop, and told me to label it and store it in a safe place? I set it on the counter, where I'd see it later and remember to ask him about it.

An hour or so later, though, my curiosity got the better of me. The container had warmed up enough by then to break the frozen seal. It looked like the beef I sometimes cooked in the crock-pot, with gravy made of coffee and onion soup mix. I sniffed; it smelled like my family's favorite roast beef in coffee sauce . . . roast beef in sauce! I looked at the label again. Sure enough, it said, "Roast Beef in Sauce."

I'm vegetarian, so I didn't taste it. But nobody in my family complained when I served it that evening. I did warn them, though:

"Let me know if any of you feels especially sparkly after you eat, or if your joints move more easily than usual." One of the girls asked, "Uh oh, another flutter, right?"

Right!

A "flutter," when we're not talking about birds, has an unofficial neurological definition: It's a cognitive problem arising from the slowing of brain waves in the temporal lobes. It manifests as one of those quirky things that everybody, MSer or not, does at one time or another. You seal the envelope and mail it to the utility company, and then discover that you forgot to enclose the check for that month's payment. You finish your cup of coffee and put the empty cup back in the china cabinet rather than in the dishwasher. You meet your next-door neighbor at the mall and can't remember his name or where you've seen him before. It's no big deal, right?

Probably not. Just ask Ron or my kids. They've gotten used to the unpredictable ways my brain works. Most of the time, they take it in stride. That's just me, right? But if they were to talk to the family of another MSer, they'd discover that it's not just me. That MSer does the same silly stuff, and so does that other one. Talk to enough MS family members, and a bizarre pattern will emerge. We all share a tendency to think, speak, write, read, and act with little deviations that, viewed individually, seem to be only minor eccentricities. Put them all together, though, and you have to wonder if we're in the middle of some kind of epidemic brain disorder. The stories all sound similar, as if we've all been bitten by the same bug, whose venom causes momentary intellectual blackouts.

We generally refer to these as "mental flutters." Or, if we happen to be in a more aristocratic mood, we call them "cerebral short-circuits." On our most down-to-earth days, they're "brain farts." The last term is, I think, the most apt. What we're talking about here is unexpected, often explosive, little outbursts of cognitive flatulence, probably brought on by emotional or intellectual intake beyond what can be comfortably digested.

They're usually along the line of the "Sally's Fridge" incident. Sally, one of the regulars in our group of online MS "flutterers," lost her TV remote control one day. After looking in all the likely spots in the house for it with no success, she finally found it in her refrigerator. Since then, "Sally's Fridge" has become a euphemism for "the most unlikely place," which is exactly the best place to look first for lost items. Anybody who loses anything at all—coffee-stained slippers, mismatched socks, car keys, checkbooks, the dog's collar—is advised to look for it in Sally's Fridge.

Here is the official description:

▲▲▲

SALLY — This is not just a fridge; it's *the* Fridge. The Official Flutterbuds' Sisterhood Fogbound Ranch Fridge, home of missing objects. It's known to come up with just about anything that drops into Sally's Place, which is that zone that absorbs whatever object you really need at the moment, and which seems to have a strange, unknown connection with Mr. Murphy of Murphy's Law fame (I'm gonna strangle that sucker if I ever catch up with him!).

Now, the Fridge's original home was the Mental Flutters Folder of the MS message boards. However, due to complaints from some unnamed individuals (who worried that the Fridge's presence there would lower property values or something like that), I picked up my Fridge and went home (so there!). It has been moved to the Fogbound Ranch [the now-imaginary/future-real—we hope—retreat for our ladies and their loved ones], where its true nature can be appreciated and enjoyed by the Sisterhood. It seems to be much happier in its new surroundings.

Much like my dog Sandy, the Fridge is a very loyal, humble, hardworking, and appreciative appliance that welcomes all of the heat-intolerant Sisterhood into its cool arms on hot days. It also tries its damnedest to come up with lost objects that need to be E-mailed back to their respective owners (assuming that our Internet servers will allow uploads of such big files). This Fridge has been responsible for rescuing, housing, and returning many items, such as blow-dryers, remote controls, brushes, pot holders, etc., belonging to many folks, most of whom are now part of the Sisterhood.

▲▲▲

Of course, some missing items still manage to turn up in likely places before they have to be relegated to Sally's Fridge. The problem is that we don't think to look there soon enough, if ever.

There have been times when I've lost some household item, spent hours looking for it, cleaned out every drawer and closet where it might lurk, and ended up not only unable to find it, but unable to remember what item I'd been looking for in the first place.

Flutters commonly involve kitchen appliances other than the refrigerator, too:

▲▲▲

JANIS — Let me just say, you cannot shut off the dumb garbage disposal with the water faucet! I tried it again last night. Guess I just couldn't remember the first time I did this, last month!

▲▲▲

JAMIE — That's okay, Janis; I still open the fridge to get my coffee when the microwave signals that it's hot!

▲▲▲

There are those of us who sniff our watches to find out what time it is (then tap the watch to see if it's still running when sniffing doesn't give us the correct information), turn on the faucet when it's too dark to see in the bathroom (then check the pipes to make sure the electricity's still on), and punch seven numbers into the calculator (eleven, if it's long distance) and wait for someone to answer (then, when nobody does, press *Clear* and try again). My own favorite flutter happened one evening when I was getting ready to brush my dogs. I sat on the floor and called Ebby to me, then picked up the TV remote control and pointed it at him. No matter how many times I flicked the on/off switch in his direction, he wouldn't lie down. I was actually getting angry at him until I realized what I was doing. I mean, I've had dogs all my life, and never once heard that a remote control is an effective command instrument.

These are the everyday occurrences that we find amusing, if occasionally a bit annoying. Sometimes, though, flutters can be frightening, especially at the beginning of MS, when it first becomes obvious that there is a definite cognitive malfunction.

I first noticed that something wasn't quite right upstairs some years after I was diagnosed with MS, when I was working for a newspaper. We had just gotten new computers at work and were going through training sessions. I was using a mouse for the first time. Our editor stood behind me and watched as I struggled to distinguish between left and right, up and down, large and small. He finally asked me if I'd ever been diagnosed as dyslexic. I turned around and looked at him to see if he was kidding. He wasn't—he looked very serious, and more than a little concerned.

Shortly after that, when I'd proofread my own work, I would find that I frequently switched around the letters in words, the words in sentences, the sentences in paragraphs, and anything else that wasn't stapled to the computer screen. That was scary; I knew I couldn't carry on a wanna-be career in journalism if I had no control over the words I wrote. It got even scarier when I tried to interview story subjects—over the phone, since by that time I'd already stopped driving. Although I was sure I could hear what they were saying, I couldn't understand it. Unless I was face-to-face with people and could watch their lips move and take note of their body language, their speech was, on first impression, indecipherable to me. It was like being in a foreign country; I'd studied the language, and so I was familiar with it, but I hadn't developed an "ear" for it. It took some time, then, for the words to sink in and make sense.

That problem continues today, with no apparent improvement even when my other symptoms are relatively quiet. To add to the fun, I now also have trouble getting understandable words to come out of my mouth. I construct in my mind exactly what I want to say. Then, when I start to speak, something very different emerges. Words that have been part of my everyday vocabulary for years come out twisted, convoluted beyond recognition. Sometimes they bear a vague resemblance to the words I originally chose, with the same beginning letter or maybe the same number of syllables. Sometimes they have roughly the meaning that I intended. At other times, the words are never-before-spoken originals, with no meaning that I can fathom and no clue as to where they came from.

Recently I made a set of pot holders for a friend who had just redecorated her kitchen. When I tried to tell another friend about them, I could only think to call them "pipe cleaners." I actually got angry because she couldn't understand what I was talking about. I knew I had the wrong words, but I couldn't find the right ones, and figured that if I knew what I was saying, she should know, too.

This brand of word substitution, as long as it's not part of formal, public communication, is one of the lighter, more interesting parts of our cognitive malfunction. One of our ladies told us about finding a family of raccoons in her back yard. When she tried to tell someone else about it, the only word she could think of for *raccoons* was "Republicans." This was during an election year, so she got some interesting comments on her slip. Another member of our group rescued an orphaned baby raccoon at about that time. We ended up adopting him as our mascot, naming him FDR (Freddie Da Raccoon) and conspiring to register him to run in the next presidential election.

The word substitution extends to reading and writing, too. One of our group told us, via E-mail, about having to "watch out for funnel clouds during a tomato warning." Another wrote back that she'd read that message as "watch out for funeral clouds during a tomato warning." Another responded further, "I hope it doesn't hail and ruin my new tornado plants!"

How about my latest one? There was an inspirational post on one of the MS bulletin boards. It ended with, "If you want humility, you must first have self-esteem." I read it as "If you want humidity, you must first self-steam." I had to double-check to make sure I hadn't stumbled onto the meteorological boards!

Then there was the discussion about what were supposed to be "love balloons" sent by Pat to one of our Sisters who wasn't feeling well:

▲▲▲

PAT — Sending my prayers, good thoughts, loafs [sic] of baboons, and gentle wishes your way.

▲▲▲

VICKI — I'm sorry. I tried to let it pass, but just couldn't. Is a loaf of baboons better than sliced bread?

▲▲▲

JAMIE — I did let it pass the first time, but I couldn't this time (I tried, I really did!). Pat, where do I go to get these "baboon loaves"? I know a few monkeys I'd like to feed!

▲▲▲

Ron recently bought me a voice recognition program for my computer that will translate my spoken words into type; I'll use it frequently and gratefully, I'm sure. I'm plagued not only by my hands going off and typing words that I'm not even thinking, but by intention tremors. This little symptom showed up as I was getting comfortably into writing this book. If I keep my hands relaxed on the keyboard and type in a steady rhythm, I do fine. But if I move either hand to grab my computer mouse or scratch my nose, my hands lose their momentum; they panic and go into an uncontrolled frenzy, twitching and jerking across the keyboard. This gets worse if I notice that I've made a typographical error and try to go back and correct it. I end up with type that's even less comprehensible than if I'd just let the mistake stand as it was.

The program will also read typewritten text to me. I don't know if I'll use that part so often, especially in conversations with the Flutterbuds. I've actually begun to let word substitution have free rein in my reading, again especially in conversations with the Flutterbuds. If the program reads exactly what's written, I may miss out on some of the fun of misreading on my own. The misreadings sometimes carry a kind of Freudian connotation; with a bit of introspection, I can use them to discern what's happening on a deeper, less obvious level of my psyche. For example, when one of our ladies writes that she's "having major trouble with this new sx" (abbreviation for *symptoms*), I read it as "having major trouble with this new sex." I might advise her, before I catch myself, to try going back to the missionary position. Likewise, if one says that her new "tx" (abbreviation for *treatment*) isn't doing any good, I might ask her when a "tax" has done anybody any good.

These are the kind of meaningless happenings that we can just let ourselves enjoy. They almost always send our group into a long, equally meaningless discussion.

And then, the program won't correct the words that just plain emerge wrong from my mouth. Sometimes I've found that even when the right word is screaming in my brain, I can't get it to come past my tongue. In the past, I was an eager conversationalist in most situations. I was comfortable speaking at meetings, teaching, doing readings in church. Now I've come to dread any but the most casual conversations in the most relaxed atmospheres. Even during phone calls with family members and close friends, it's better if I just concentrate on what the other person is saying, while keeping my own side of the conversation to a minimum. It really is too much to handle the input and output at the same time. I wonder how many potential friendships I've squelched, or how many established friendships I've ruined, by my seeming unwillingness to communicate.

It became obvious a long time ago that this whole scenario involves more than just an occasional, momentary mental slip. It's more like an ongoing mental flub-up, one that lingers for much longer than a moment. It's what we call "MS Fog." Thus the name for our dream-resort, Fogbound Ranch, where it will be perfectly acceptable, safe, dignified, and normal to wander around with our heads in a perpetual mist.

Seriously, though, before I learned to laugh with the others at our flutters, I worried that something was terribly wrong with the way my brain worked. I caught myself looking into the future and seeing myself a slobbering, babbling fool, destined to wander through the rest of my life completely unaware of my own disintegration. The most annoying part has been that, even when I manage to say something intelligible, my short-term memory goes on vacation, and I end up repeating the same thing two or three times before I realize that the people around me have heard it before.

The neurologist I saw years ago when this all started told me that mental difficulties weren't associated with multiple sclerosis. I asked him to test me for Alzheimer's, dyslexia, brain tumors, or whatever else might be wrong. He did a CAT scan, which was normal, and then said I was probably just stressed and that I should relax. It wasn't until several years later that another neurologist (the one I see now) told me that, yes, MS can cause impaired mental function. All MS problems are related to the central nervous system's inability to smoothly send and carry signals to other parts of the body. It's only logical that signals heading out to facilitate comprehension and other abstract processes will also hit some detours along the way. Dr. R. went on to assure me that this aspect of MS rarely progresses to full dementia. That's when I relaxed, at least a little.

Even with assurance from a knowledgeable doctor that these symptoms are par for the course and rarely cause for worry, MSers can't avoid the real fear, at least in the beginning, that their brains are turning to oatmeal. Just how far can this kind of mental dysfunction extend?

I've read a lot on the subject, and I have concluded that there's no scientific way to measure the extent of this problem. There are means of determining that some cognitive changes usually take place in the course of MS progression. Like many aspects of MS, cognitive impairment, and the manners in which it manifests itself in the disease, vary considerably from one MSer to another. Clinical tests frequently can't account for the differences. An MRI might show lesions, which may or may not be located in areas of the brain that correspond to the cognitive symptoms being experienced. One exam might indicate that a person with MS has gone through a certain measure of cognitive changes. Another exam, or the person's subjective comprehension of the changes, may indicate malfunction on a much higher or lower level.

Sometimes, when it seems that one of the Flutterbuds has locked into an especially clearheaded, flutter-free interval, a bigger flutter is actually lurking beneath the surface. For instance, when our group was in the initial stages of formation, Renee came up with the idea of all of us Sisters keeping in touch by means of round-robin letters—each of us would write one or two long letters every day, enclosing little blurbs for each member within those letters. Then we would post the letters to everyone in our group. It was a well-organized plan to cut down on one-liner clutter in our E-mailboxes. But the simple formula, thought up by Renee to help her avoid fluttering through her E-mail, itself turned into a monumental flutter for her. She often had to repeat to herself (and to us) the mechanics of her own plan, so that she could remember how to follow through with it:

▲▲▲

RENEE — Okay, when I use round robin in the subject area, I am saying, "This is to everyone." Okay? You see, lately I can't figure out exactly what is happening. I just know that if I change anything within my routine, my brain acts like a brat and refuses to accept information. I'm as serious as a heart attack! Like, if I want to send something to one of you, if I put "To ____," which I don't normally use, everything after that is off-kilter and so confusing that I have to just give up. I come up with so many typos and word substitutions, I can't believe it. Sometimes I see something I wrote and it has all these strange words where they don't belong.

So I'm trying. For the time being, I'm just going to try to stick with one letter with blurbs to everyone. Sorry, all of you who came up with other wonderful ideas on how to curtail some of this mail. I will try to keep my blurbs brief. Brief blurbs! Brief blurbs! Say that ten times real fast!

▲▲▲

All of us have complained about how our memories frequently desert us, with no warning, no rhyme or reason; they just decide to take a vacation. The forgotten facts are most likely to be things previously (and, we thought, permanently) etched on the most conscious areas of our brains.

▲▲▲

DONNA — Once, on a business trip, I had the most horrible experience with remembering. I went shopping and found a really neat sale. When I went to purchase the items, I saw that I didn't have my credit card (it was at home in another purse), so I paid with the cash I had on me, since I had seen an ATM machine on my way to the mall. I used the last of my folding money on dinner and headed back to the hotel, stopping at the ATM on the way.

I *could not* remember my number—just four little digits. I could remember that it was a significant date in my life, but not the significance. The bank only gives you six tries before it takes your card and makes you go through a humiliation ritual to get the thing back. I didn't know this at the time, so when I entered the sixth series of numbers and the machine started rumbling, I thought *bingo!* Wrong. All I got was a piece of paper telling me to contact my bank, 150 miles away, on the next business day to get the card back.

I had a couple of dollars in change and less than a quarter of a tank of gas; I was in a strange town 150 miles from home and did not want to admit my stupidity to anyone. I did what any intelligent, resourceful person would do—I called my husband, crying. He saved the day by wiring me the money to make it home, with a little extra to salve my bruised ego, and he never mentioned it again. Memories like that remind me of how nice it is to have a significant other to bail you out when you need bailing out. I also haven't forgotten the number again, and wrote it in telephone-number format on everything I could think of.

▲▲▲

It's not all bad. Helen reminds us that the forgetfulness part of fluttering does have an up side:

— When we hear a joke, we never have to interrupt the teller with "I've heard that one";

— The rerun season on TV is as entertaining as the first-run season;

— We never get tired of eating leftovers;

— We can read the same book or watch the same movie over and over and never get bored;

— We can hide our own Easter baskets!

I've discovered another, very real, benefit to this aspect of the MS battle. While my short-term memory has crumbled, my long-term memory seems to have improved. If I hear a song from the '60s or '70s or get a whiff of a cologne that was popular back in those days, I don't just remember; I'm transported back there.

The odd thing about this is that I've seen medical reports about cognitive problems in MS that claim that short-term memory remains intact while long-term recall disintegrates. I have to strongly disagree with that pronouncement. We haven't discussed this in much detail within our group, but I know that others have had experiences similar to mine, which contradict that idea. Sometimes when we're chatting, one or another of us will slip in a reference to something (a movie, a song or a songwriter, a dance, an article of clothing) that was popular twenty or thirty (or forty!) years ago. All other discussion stops immediately, and the computer screen is flooded with reports of the memories that are surging back to each of us. If one of us mentions occasions we experienced way back when, proms or Scout campouts or even kindergarten field trips, we can all remember the clothes we wore on our own similar days, the foods we ate at those events, and the names of all the people who were with us at those times. We might not be so popular anymore in the minds of the people with whom we forgot another appointment. But the popularity level rises when it's time to play nostalgia trivia games!

▲▲▲

LORI — It's so funny; this subject comes up here quite frequently. My husband is eleven years older than I am (he's thirty-nine), yet he almost never gets any music trivia questions right, and I usually do. He gets so mad. It might be okay if we could blame it on drugs or something, but he never did any. For some reason, I have a huge capacity for totally worthless trivia—not the trivia that can win you lots of money on *Jeopardy*, but trivia about songs and artists, television shows and actors, who they were back then, theme songs to movies that are used over and over for other movies. I just pick up on stuff like that. I have no idea why. I would much rather be able to simply remember where I put my keys, thank you!

▲▲▲

Some of these mental gaps, though, do go beyond funny, annoying, or embarrassing, and head right up to dangerous. Like leaving a candle burning on the wooden dining table or forgetting that it's not a good idea to stick your hand into the garbage disposal while it's running.

I had one of these incidents after I'd already given up driving. It was at a time when I felt pretty good and considered getting back behind the wheel. One evening Ron and I went to the grocery store. We took along my electric scooter, which I used regularly on shopping trips. We crossed the parking lot and I gave the scooter an extra burst of power to get up the little ramp at the entrance to the store. At that point, I realized that the automatic doors were not working properly; they were opening much too slowly to allow me to get through safely. I knew I had to stop or at least slow down, a maneuver that required only a flick of my thumb on the control lever. But I couldn't remember how to do it! I could only sit there and watch my reflection in the glass come rapidly closer. Luckily, Ron was able to grab the seat and slow the scooter down enough to prevent a serious crash. I've never again even thought about trying to drive a real car, out there on real roads, with real people in the vicinity.

I'm one of the lucky ones. Others have had closer calls.

▲▲▲

PAT — Having survived my first serious multiple sclerosis attack, involving more than a year in a wheelchair, physical therapy for pain, weeks on crutches, and all the other scary stuff, I thought I pretty much had a handle on this MS thing.

Then came my first "major" mental flutter. One day, after an exhausting food-shopping excursion with my six-year-old daughter, I paid for the groceries and headed out of the store. Just as I approached the exit, three security guards stepped out of nowhere and shuffled me off into a small room. There, behind a large desk, sat a man surrounded by TV monitors that showed the entire store. "Do you shoplift often?" he asked. Shoplift? What was he talking about? I had just paid for $150 worth of groceries! One of the guards lifted up my purse, which I'd put in the top of the food cart. Underneath it sat some make-up items I'd picked up. "Oh, my, I forgot all about that," I started to explain.

"That's not what the camera shows," I was told. The man then showed me a tape of myself on the monitor, looking around the store and fumbling with my purse and the cart at the same time. I must admit it did look a little odd, but I explained that I'd just been looking around for my daughter. No one believed me.

"Sign this paper admitting to the theft and you can leave. But you can't come into this store again. We don't cater to shoplifters!"

Shoplifter? What was going on? All this over a few dollars' worth of cosmetics? All of a sudden I went brain dead. The "mental flutters" had set in. I was being badgered to sign the paper or go to jail. I was too shocked to defend myself. The more the guards threatened, the worse I became. I forgot about my daughter, still out in the store somewhere. I didn't know what to do or say. I couldn't even think.

Finally, I was told I could make one phone call. "My husband," I muttered. Later, while waiting for him to come and get me, I began to feel weak. My vision blurred, and numbness and tingling sensations migrated down my right side. Signs of a real exacerbation were beginning, but I couldn't even comprehend that. My brain had turned into oatmeal.

When my husband arrived, the guards told him of my "crime." He tried to explain about my illness, the forgetfulness, etc.

"She signs the paper or goes to jail," the guards repeated.

My husband could see that my condition was getting worse. Anxious to get me away from there, he told me to sign the paper. I did. As we left the store, he had to hold onto me to keep me from falling. I was a wreck!

As we drove home, my husband asked who was watching our daughter. Our daughter! She wasn't with us! What had I done now? We went back to the store, and my husband found her happily walking the food aisles, not the least bit aware of all that had happened.

But I was aware . . . aware that this MS had totally screwed up my brain! Why wasn't I able to defend myself? Where was the quick wit I once had? Why did I "lose it"? Why did I sign those papers? How could I forget my own daughter? I was terrified of the answers to those questions.

After that, it took a long time to get over the fear of going out alone. Would I be able to manage on my own? Would my children be safe with me? I struggled with these and many other concerns. I began to work "safety features" into my life. I kept track of everything I'd bought or intended to buy. I never let my children out of my sight, no matter what. I kept a list of phone numbers of people to call in case of a mental flutter. My motto became, "If in doubt, call for help."

For a long time after this incident, I made a lot of those calls for help. Sometimes the reasons were urgent. Other times not. To this day, I still call for help, although many times, by the time help arrives, I've forgotten why I called! My confidence is slowly returning, although I know now that the mental flutters will remain an ever-present part of my MS fight.

▲▲▲

I don't know of any medication that is supposed to clear brain fog. Some MSers have found that increased mental alertness is a side effect of medications they take for other reasons. For instance, some antidepressants can increase alertness. While I was on Amantadine for fatigue, I could think a bit more clearly. I heard a news report lately that said that daily supplements of vitamin E can improve mental function. That might be true; I've been taking it every day for the past six months for menopausal symptoms, and my flutters do seem to have slowed. But, as with treatment of any MS symptom, there's no proof that sharper mental acuity results directly from any medication or supplement, that it is an added benefit of improved overall well-being, or that it simply marks the remission of a single MS symptom.

It does help (and this has been proven) to spend time in activities that call for quick, logical thinking. It's the old "exercise improves function" truism. I play solitaire games on the computer to sharpen my mind (well, it's a good excuse, anyway, to just play every day).

Mostly, however, we depend on our own experience to help us forestall the effects of our flutters. We know that we must:

— Set timers to remind ourselves that we have food in the oven, the hose running in the garden, or children to be picked up at school; to take a pill; or do anything else that requires our attention at a particular moment. Then we have to write notes to remind ourselves why we set the timers.

— Accept the fact that our homes, offices, and vehicles hereafter all will have hundreds of little sticky yellow notepapers as a major part of their decor. A good supply of these notes, scattered abundantly through the areas we frequent, reminds us what to do. We should also remember to read notes to ourselves twice before taking any action.

That's the best way to avoid using roast beef in sauce to prevent rust buildup on appliances!

— Ask at least one other person to remind us one hour before we have any kind of appointment (helpful even when a timer has been set).

— Keep how-to-operate instructions *forever* for all appliances and mechanical items in our homes. (After using my sewing machine at least 5,000 times, I've had to sit down and figure out, one more time, how to thread it. I've also, at various times, forgotten how to turn on the dishwasher, the vacuum cleaner, my stereo, and the front porch light.)

— Not obsess over our inability to program the VCR, set the time on the new alarm clock, or learn a game on the computer—no matter how detailed the instructions.

— When following a recipe, line up all ingredients on the counter at the very beginning. Then put each away as it is added in the correct measure to the others. Otherwise, cultivate a taste for very spicy chili, very stiff biscuits, and very moist cakes. There's just no other way to avoid the consequences of forgetting that you've already added the red peppers, the flour, or the water. Another hint: Before starting to cook, clear the counter of anything that shouldn't end up in your recipe. Like the spray bottle of antibacterial kitchen cleaner (instead of the butter-flavored cooking spray) that I once picked up to coat the tortillas I was using to make quesadillas.

— Not be embarrassed about wearing a shirt inside out or backward.

— When all else fails, check Sally's Fridge!

6

Family Matters

LORI — Today was not a good day. It was Amanda's [Lori's six-year-old daughter] first day of school. I'm not sad about that; I've gotten used to the idea of her being away at school, as we have had her in different programs already. What got me was when she looked at me as we were leaving and said, "Mom, you're not gonna bring *that,* are you?" (referring to my cane). "The kids will laugh at you and you will look. . . ." She stopped.

"I will look what?" I asked.

"I can't say it, it's a bad word."

"What letter does it start with?"

"S."

"I will look stupid?" I finished for her.

"Yes," she replied. "I don't want the kids to laugh at you."

I can understand where she's coming from, but today that hurt me so deep down. It's not anything I can change. It's not anything I can make all better or make go away. I can't fix it. I am an embarrassment. My daughter is ashamed of me.

Why isn't this something I can fix? We all want to make the lives of our children easier than what we went through, but I don't even have a chance with this one.

Don't get me wrong. I am not going through the "why me's," and I totally understand Amanda's feelings. I know she did not mean to hurt me with her words. It's just one of those situations that smacks you full upside your head (and heart) and makes you stop dead in your tracks, completely breathless. I guess I don't like surprises much anymore. Yes, I am a little depressed. I think that is to be expected, but I will be all right.

I am all out of tears now, but I have plenty of saltwater taffy and marshmallows to get me through (no damn chocolate to be found anywhere!).

▲▲▲

It's one thing to expect (and get!) a variety of reactions from those around us when we start to use canes and other assistive devices. (Chapter Six talks about how we handle that.) It's another story, though, when the reactions come from members of our own families. It's especially painful to hear something like this from one of our children, and even worse when the child is as young as Amanda. Something inside us rips apart when this happens. We know instinctively that the child's worry is not just that Mom will be laughed at or "look stupid." We're all too aware that, hidden behind the mask of simple embarrassment, is anger that something bad has happened to "*my* mom." There's hurt because the child feels deprived of a mom "like all the other kids' moms." There's raw fear that the "something bad" will turn into something worse, so much worse that the child can't name it.

We in the Froup are lucky that we're all at different stages in raising our children. It's a comfort to be able to run to our computers and talk, right that minute, to other MS moms about the repercussions our disease has on our innocent little ones. It's truly lifesaving to have somebody like Sharon available, somebody who can look at the scene objectively and offer understanding and practical advice.

▲▲▲

Lori, Amanda's feelings about your cane are a very age-appropriate response. I can understand how much it hurt you. My own daughter (fourteen years old) is embarrassed by my tremor and my limp. Because of her age, though, I am able to use the opportunity to teach her that people with disabilities are not any different on the inside. They have feelings just like she does, and like everybody else who doesn't have physical problems.

Anything at all different is cause for kids to feel embarrassed or to lash out or to laugh. My kids' school brings in puppets and people with disabilities so that the children can experience what it's like to be in a wheelchair or to be blind or deaf. Just last year, my twelve-year-old came home from school and told me that a group like this came into her classroom. As part of their demonstration, they asked her to tie on a blindfold and count out change from a desk. Then she had to put her right hand behind her and try to read a book with one hand. She had to try to wheel a chair into a tiny bathroom stall, and to open the heavy front door of the school while sitting in the chair. When she came home that afternoon, she told me she knew what it was like for me. I asked her how she felt about that, and she began to cry. She has been most helpful since that program!

Our children want and need us to be perfect. But it becomes our job to guide and respectfully direct them toward the unfortunate realities in life, like multiple sclerosis.

We can't do anything about our disease, and our kids know that. Amanda is just a little girl who loves you so much that it hurts her to see you with that cane. It hurts her that her peers might laugh at you.

I'm sorry that you had to experience this, Lori, but it was bound to happen eventually. As our children get older, they are more exposed to the cruelties of life. I have found that children can be a really tough bunch and, at the same time, a really loving bunch. This is an opportunity to teach Amanda how to live with her own emotions about the situation around her, and to still be proud of her mom. As she matures, it will get easier for

Hunter House is your publisher for books about

| health and wellness especially women's health | personal growth and sexuality | domestic violence and teen violence | resources for counselors and educators on
 • violence prevention
 • trauma in children |

Hunter House

Books for health, family and community

☐ To receive a copy of our latest catalog please check this box and return this card. Please circle the categories you are most interested in.

We are looking for a few good authors.

If you are a writer with expertise in the areas we publish, we want to see your manuscript. Call for our guidelines or e-mail us at: acquisitions@hunterhouse.com

BOOK IN WHICH THIS CARD WAS FOUND (Please print)

NAME

ORGANIZATION

ADDRESS

CITY   STATE   ZIP OR POSTAL CODE   COUNTRY (if not USA)

I WOULD LIKE TO SEE A BOOK PUBLISHED ABOUT

order Hunter House books call toll-free 1-800-266-5592
ail: ordering@hunterhouse.com   Web site: www.hunterhouse.com

HUNTER HOUSE INC., PUBLISHERS
Mailing List
P.O. Box 2914
Alameda CA 94501-0914

her to say, "My mom has MS and she uses a cane to help her walk and I love her."

▲▲▲

LORI — Thanks for your support about what happened with Amanda. I knew she was not being hurtful. It's as I said, just another of those things that comes up and smacks you upside the head. Several people have mentioned getting in touch with the school or the teacher and suggesting that they have a presentation on differently-abled people. I think this is a marvelous idea and will pursue it once things calm down and the kids are more settled in their classes and with one another. I think it is something that I do not want to be an active part of, though. That might put Amanda in the spotlight too much, and she is not very good at that. I know of a few programs here that go around to schools and educate, so I think I will solicit help from them.

[Later] Well, I'm still all for educating our kids about the problems of people with disabilities. But now that we've had a chance to talk about it, I don't think it's an urgent requirement for Amanda. She told me this afternoon that she wants me to take my cane tomorrow so the other kids can see it. She said she was really worried this morning that they would laugh at me, because they didn't know about "canes and that kind of stuff." But now she has explained to them that I have MS, and that that means I'm "talented." I asked her how she'd figured that out. She said that being talented means having "extra gifts, things that most other people don't have." Since most other people don't have MS, then I must be talented!

▲▲▲

JANE — We have three children, who were all born after my diagnosis. I have been fortunate that my MS remained mild and I had mostly invisible symptoms while they were small.

They knew Mommy's legs got tired easily, that I sometimes limped, that I napped more than most mommies. When they were older, they learned that the heat was bad for me, so I maybe couldn't make it to every one of their ball games. They knew that there were times when I wasn't quite up to whatever they wanted me to do, but I never told them that this was because I had multiple sclerosis.

When our eldest child was a senior in high school, I decided I wanted him to know. That way, he would have a whole year to see me getting along just fine before he went off to college in another state. He felt a little funny that we hadn't told him before, because we are a very honest, straightforward family on absolutely everything else. Yet he did see my reasoning and agreed that it had prevented a lot of problems. He did not feel deceived. He understood our belief that there wasn't anything the children could have done about the situation, so there was no reason to threaten their security by telling them about it. This, of course, would not be my recommendation to everyone else, but it was right for us under the circumstances. Since my MS was benign, I thought the knowledge of my diagnosis would be harder on everybody than the actual disease would be.

We told the other two children individually in the following years, and they had similar reactions. Now, the impact of all these years of hiding the MS has been mainly on me. I have essentially borne the burden of the disease behind closed doors with my husband, so to speak. But I am still very glad that the children were able to live a totally normal childhood, unburdened by unnecessary fear of the future. I always said that as long as I didn't have to be hospitalized, I'd stick to my decision. I've been fortunate to have the less aggressive (although totally obnoxious and painful) kind of MS.

▲▲▲

BREN — Here's a cute one for y'all. Yesterday, Kristy came in from school and told me she'd been dropping stuff all day in her class: pencils, pens, paper, etc. So I sympathized with her, and then sent her to do her chores. In the space of two minutes, she dropped my return-address label holder three times. Every time, she managed to pick it up only to drop it again. I chuckled and told her to take it in the kitchen to put in the cabinet. She headed to the kitchen, where she tripped over the phone, dropped the receiver on the floor when she tried to pick it up, and then dropped the labels again in the kitchen.

From the kitchen, I heard this frustrated yell: "Mom! I've got MS!"

Well, I spewed diet Coke all over the place. I hugged her and told her that she most probably doesn't have MS, but that I knew how frustrating all the dropping had been that day. Then we had a good laugh about it all, and she felt better.

▲▲▲

I don't remember having any discussions with my kids about multiple sclerosis per se when they were small. They were aware that I had it; they'd heard the adults in the family refer to it often enough. They were just toddlers when I was diagnosed, so they kind of grew up with the knowledge that their mom was a bit different from most other moms. (I guess they would have come to that conclusion even if I didn't have MS!) They knew that the difference was somehow the result of Mom's "EM ESS." But that awareness was relative, I think, and varied depending on how the disease affected me (and them) at any given moment. They weren't aware that Mom's little difference could get much larger in the future.

During their childhoods, I, like Jane, was fortunate enough to have mostly mild attacks followed by long periods of remission. I managed to keep up with most of the other mothers, helping out in school activities, leading a Girl Scout troop, and chauffeuring the girls and their friends to other activities. It just wasn't a big deal that my girls' mom was sick once in a while. After all, didn't the other mothers get colds and have to stay home from school events, or sprain their ankles and have to use crutches to get around, or even have problems that sent them to the hospital for a few days?

It was only when they got older, in high school and college, that Karen and Julie reacted visibly to my illness (which was also the time that my MS turned progressive). Then it was hard, I admit, to interpret their reactions. I kind of regretted then that we hadn't treated the MS as a more significant presence in our lives.

Karen left home for college and expressed worries about being unable to be with me when I was sick. Julie sometimes found it too painful to be at home, where she had to watch as my condition deteriorated. Those responses were apparent; whatever else was going on in their minds and hearts, however, is still pretty much a mystery to me.

I realize that I made another big mistake while the girls were growing up (one that, regrettably, I continue to make today). I have sent and do send mixed messages to all my family and close friends, but especially to my daughters. I tell them that I'm fine, and then resent them when I feel that they expect too much of me. When Karen offers, during her visits home, to walk the dogs, I insist that walking the dogs is a point of pride for me, that I have to do it even when it's almost impossible. Then I gripe, sometimes aloud and sometimes to myself, that nobody in the family can even pick up a couple of leashes, hook them to the dogs, and walk a block or two with them. They'd rather see me stagger down the street with a leash twisted around each of my crutches, a dog straining at each leash. If Julie offers to take me shopping or to a movie, I usually tell her that I'm too tired. Then I moan and groan about my cabin fever. If she decides to clean the bathroom for me, I get bitchy because she's interrupting my rest with her noise or because I know I'd be able to do a better job of it myself. Then when she goes quietly off to pursue her own interests, I accuse her of not caring that I can't manage all the housework alone anymore.

I asked the girls if they would each give me a short account of their feelings about having a parent with a chronic illness. Julie declined; she said it was too personal. Karen, though, offered this:

▲▲▲

I'm supposed to write something about how my mom's struggle with multiple sclerosis has affected me, or how I feel about it. I can't remember a time when I didn't know my mom was/would be somehow disabled, so there's almost too much to say. I have gone through feelings ranging from embarrassment to guilt to a strange sense of loss. I have been angry at various people and at the disease itself for depriving my youthful, creative, brilliant mother of the ability to enjoy even some of the most mundane pleasures.

The aspect of my mom's illness that has affected me most, I think, is the unpredictability. It's a horrible surprise to call home from a vacation in Florida only to have my sister tell me I can't talk to Mom because she's in the hospital. The greatest difficulty lies in not knowing what comes next, from the bouts of numbness and paralysis to the anxiety we all feel at the prospect of losing precious parts of Mom's personality as she progresses through the disease.

We can't even know if my sister and I are also likely to someday be diagnosed with multiple sclerosis. There's supposed to be some kind of familial tendency toward the disease, but even that is unpredictable.

My family's efforts to deal with the disease are, needless to say, trivial in comparison with what my mom must face every day. Her handwriting has changed; her appetite varies; her energy level sometimes plummets without warning; she can be downright grumpy—it is hard to love someone and see them suffer. I see my dad and sister deal with it in their particular ways. I deal with it by living my life, as my mom insists I should; but I hate the guilt I feel about living far away from her, too far to help with the little things, too far to know any more than what she tells me about how she's really feeling. But I can observe the frustration on her face when she can't remember why she came into a room. Her pride and persistence both infuriate and inspire me.

▲▲▲

The following letter is another daughter's view of having a mom with MS. It's from Joy's daughter, Jen. She, like Karen, is a young adult and lives far from her mother's home.

▲▲▲

I remember how scared I was, taking Mom around for her first batch of tests when we were trying to get a diagnosis. I realized that the time had come when I had to help my mom as opposed to the other way around. That is a terrible realization for a child (even a child twenty-five years old).

I don't claim to fully understand this illness, and I imagine that I was as unsympathetic as everybody else when we first began to deal with it. I couldn't understand why my mother couldn't drive herself to work or why she needed to take a nap on the floor of her office. I would attribute it to her not *wanting* to work, rather than to any disease. But as we learned more about MS and its debilitating symptoms, I became more defensive of her. When her boss was rude to her and totally unsympathetic, I remember wanting to call her up (Mom's boss) and give her a piece of my mind.

It's hard telling my friends, when they ask, that my mother has never been out to visit me here in California. They don't understand that it is not because she doesn't want to; it's because she isn't able to. And it saddens me to think of all the things that we will miss out on because of her disease. That includes the realization that she may never make it out here, even if I settle here and have a family. I know that she is a victim of MS. But I think we are all victims, because it robs us of quality time with our loved ones.

▲▲▲

Most of the ladies in our group have children who are at least old enough to understand the significance of having a mom with a chronic, potentially disabling illness. Ramia's kids are, I think, the youngest of our members' offspring:

▲▲▲

My kids, ages two and six, are really too young to "get it." Brian did the MS Walk [an annual fundraising event for the National Multiple Sclerosis Society] last spring, on Dad's shoulders half the time. Haley did it in the stroller, with me pushing. Brian has seen his dad give me my Avonex shot; he just sort of takes it in stride. He can't understand why I get tired every afternoon and just don't have energy to do things with his sister and himself. That makes me pretty damn mad also, because being tired makes me the bitch from hell! Just thinking about it makes me mad.

▲▲▲

MY RESPONSE — Gee, Momia Ramia, it seems to me that you're doing a pretty good job of helping your kids to "get it." You're not shoving it in their faces every day, but you let them see that you have a hard time functioning on some days, you show them how you're doing whatever you can medically to help yourself, and you're letting them be involved in the long-term aspect of "doing something about it." They probably "get it" more than we, or even they, realize.

▲▲▲

We recognize, of course, that multiple sclerosis has an impact on family members other than just our children. I've tried to discern how other members of my family feel about the whole deal. I don't want to put them on the spot by asking them directly. I guess I can only judge by the overt signals I've gotten over the years.

My father died long before I was diagnosed with MS, so he fortunately never had to know about it. Mom was affected deeply, I know. She asked me several times if I knew of anything that she'd done that might have caused me to get the illness. She was always more than willing to step in whenever I needed help with anything, and she worried constantly about me doing things like going up and down steps to do the laundry or going for a walk out of sight of whomever I was with at the time. That was all characteristic of Mom's concern for each of her kids. The only peculiar thing I noticed was that each time I had to be hospitalized for treatment during the last few years before her death in 1993, she came up with some excuse not to visit me there. I was hurt at the time, but looking back I realize that she just didn't want me to see how upset she was.

I have to admit that, since Mom died, there have been several times when I was disturbingly relieved, almost happy, that she wasn't alive anymore. I've missed her every single minute since she left, but I'm so grateful that she hasn't had to witness the more rapid deterioration of my health in these past few years.

My siblings (Joyce, Ruth, and Sandy; and Jim, who died in 1996) have supported and helped as much as I've allowed them to. They, along with my mom, took over whenever I couldn't mother my girls adequately. I'm thankful that I no longer have to ask them for that kind of help. I'll accept their offers of a ride (if one of them happens to be going to the same place that I'm going) or their assistance with hosting a family party. But I can't bring myself to ask them for favors if they don't offer first, and most times even if they do offer. The same goes for my friends Donna and Sis. I accept Donna's rides to our dentist twice a year and to the radiologist for our mammograms once a year, and Sis is very helpful about providing a way to club meetings and school performances. Other than that, my friends and family all treat me as if I'm not in any way "handicapped," and that's the way I prefer it.

Then, of course, there's my husband, Ron. He offered to write something that would describe how he feels about my MS and how he deals with it as my spouse. Then I found a copy of a letter he'd sent to a friend of his at work, right after her brother was diagnosed with MS. I think it describes his feelings and dealings accurately. It also says a lot about the kind of guy he is. With his permission, I'm including it here.

▲▲▲

Dear B.,

I spent the whole evening last Thursday wondering what was responsible for the grave look on your face when I picked up my paycheck that afternoon. Your words, "I need to talk to you about MS," didn't really hit me until I was in the car on the way home. I thought of all kinds of possibilities: B. has been diagnosed with MS; M. [her husband] has been diagnosed with MS; someone really dear and close has been diagnosed.

Then you told me on Friday that F. [her brother] had been recently diagnosed with multiple sclerosis. The fact that it is your brother, as opposed to you or M., makes this news no less distressing to me. When we were told that Lynn has MS, it took quite a long time for me to accept it and to decide to make the best of a condition I wouldn't wish on my worst enemy. The disease itself is often easier to live with than the emotional and social problems that go along with it. I only pray that F.'s family will actually be drawn closer as a result of his diagnosis, just as Lynn and I have been.

As I said the other day, keeping a positive attitude is vital to the well-being of your brother and everyone around him. That will sometimes do more than any so-called wonder drug.

Remember, except in extreme departures from the norm, multiple sclerosis is a disease you die *with*, not *from*. I am in no way trying to make light of the severe impact MS has on a person's emotional and physical health. What I am trying to do is let you know that this is not the end of the world. We can, in good faith, hope that F. will soon go into remission and remain there until he dies of old age.

I'd like to emphasize that I, Lynn, and the whole network of people in the MS family are there if you or F. and his friends and family need us. I've enclosed a couple of pamphlets about MS. Should you or F. need more, contact me or the MS Society.

▲▲▲

Of course, Ron doesn't say what I know to be true: that his path to acceptance has been a rocky one, with a lot of twists and turns and ups and downs. There have been times when his actions have shouted, much louder than his words could, that he is in our marriage for the long haul, no matter how much the MS has tried to throw us off the track. When I was first diagnosed, he came to the hospital with a diamond ring for me. From that day forward, he has never given me reason to fear that he would bail out of our marriage. He has taken over each of my responsibilities as I've become unable to perform them myself. He has done everything in his power to lift me and carry me, both literally and figuratively, through our life together.

That's not to say that he doesn't need a break now and then. There have been times when I've watched him search for ways to avoid being with me. Sometimes he gets lost in his work, other times in his hobbies. Sometimes he thinks of a dozen things he has to go out and buy, at eleven different stores, in seven different counties. Even then, I know for sure that I have only to dial his pager number, and he'll drop whatever he's doing and come home.

For the past three years, Ron has been very involved in the fundraising walk sponsored by the National Multiple Sclerosis

Society, which is held every spring. He spends a good six months of every year organizing a team of walkers, soliciting individual and corporate sponsors, leading his team through the actual walk, collecting sponsorships, tracking the returns of his team members, and then sending written thanks to his walkers. Sometimes his work on this project takes up every minute of his spare time for weeks on end. I think it's good, though, because his efforts provide him with a battlefield on which to carry out his own fight against the MonSter (his team's name is, in fact, the MonSter Slayers). His involvement blunts some of the helplessness he feels as we face the Beast every day. Just as importantly, I think, it gives him a valid reason to go off to his own space and do something constructive away from the immediate presence of the MonSter. I understand that he occasionally needs his space, even though he would never say that to me.

More than anything else, I'm truly amazed and grateful that Ron is still so obviously committed to me and to us. He has put up with a lot of hell on my account ever since the MonSter showed up as the third spouse in our marriage.

Renee's husband, Burt, has much to say about the challenges of loving and living with a person with MS:

▲▲▲

What gets me is that sometimes my brain feels squeezed. When Renee has to stay in bed or stay at home because of an MS problem, she graciously tells me to go on without her and do what was planned. She tells me that the MS shouldn't control both of our lives, keep us both trapped in the house. I ride a motorcycle, and she can't ride anymore. So I go on out, ride with a group of friends, maybe ten, twenty motorcycles.

Now when you have that many people, the guys have their girls riding with them. Not me. So when I ride, sometimes I feel sad. Sad because Renee can't go. Sad because she's stuck in the house while I'm out riding, doing the things men and women do together, except that I'm doing them by myself. Sometimes I get mad. Not at Renee, but at the fucking disease. It has stripped her of so much, and us of what we used to do together.

Renee has had MS for thirteen years. We have been through the ups and downs. We've laughed together and cried together. Been the whole route. We love each other. Divorce is not an option. I just feel squeezed sometimes, frustrated. I want to do what other couples do.

Renee is a brave girl. She works hard, tries her best to make it easier for me. She has lost a lot of herself. But she keeps on keepin' on. Gives me strength.

But I still feel squeezed sometimes. It's the little things, I think, that bother me. Can't go here, can't go there. Cancel this, cancel that. Wash the clothes, go pick up a prescription at the drugstore. No more backpacking together, no more climbing the mountain.

She complains very little. Fights the Beast with humor. She's full of humor. She has a life made up of different things like art and her group of MS friends on the Internet.

Meanwhile, I go out by myself. Married, doing things other couples do, with other couples, but by myself. I feel guilty, squeezed. She didn't ask for this. She is the kind of person every caregiver should get to be with. I love her; I hate the disease.

My single friends try to hook up with a lady. I don't, but I feel awkward just sitting there while the game goes on. I'm married, but alone. I hate this disease.

There ought to be a way that all caregivers can get together, do things, go places. Men and women together, platonic friends, sharing, understanding one another's needs. Then go home, back to our spouses. Kind of like a fill-up. Pull up to the pumps of life. Fill 'er up, please. I'll take a couple gallons of doing things together. . . . Make that unguilted, please.

I've worked hard on being a good caregiver. Renee has

worked hard on coping. We hate the disease, the MonSter, who's trying to suck the nectar of life out of both of us.

Fuck you, Beast! Get out of our lives! But you hide. You make us think you've gone away, then you rear your ugly head. Cancel this. Can't do that. Renee doesn't like it any more than I do. But she tells me to go on without her. Maybe she's my caregiver. I believe that's it. She helps me cope, gently nudges me along. "Live your life. Do this. Do that. Go on, have a good time." I go, but it's hard to not be squeezed. I feel two emotions: relief that I can go, guilt for going.

Now all you college psychologists, don't tell me to work on this or work on that. Reality is real. I am working on it. Renee helps me work on living my life. We fight the Beast together.

▲▲▲

Here are ways that others have experienced family reactions to life with multiple sclerosis:

▲▲▲

CHRIS — Well, I went to the neurologist today, and I told him how I get so tired and lose my balance when I have to do a lot of walking. He said to use a cane at those times. I told him that my family wouldn't understand that. He said that it's hard to make other people understand why you need a cane, since the tiredness and loss of balance are usually invisible problems of MS.

When I came home and told my family that the doctor wants me to use a cane, the first response of some of them was, "What for?" I also told them what the doctor said about others not understanding because they can't always see that I'm tired or off-balance. They ended up just dropping the subject, but we are going to have to talk about it sometime.

▲▲▲

DEE — Chris, I really feel for you and with you about some of your family not understanding how we feel or what we can't do. I think it may have to do with control. The people who love us have no control over this disease. Still, they want everything to be as it was before the MS hit. Some nights when I go to bed, I pray that for a short time I will have some dramatic, visible change, so that other people will understand. Of course, I'd rather just go back to how I was before, or even better, but this would be just to make a point. I even feel that sometimes other people think I'm making up all my problems.

I don't have any advice for you, because I don't even know what to do in my own situation. But I will keep you in my prayers and hopes that somehow things will get better for you in this area.

▲▲▲

We all encounter times when family members don't understand how we feel or are unable to accept that we need help to move around. This problem isn't something that we can resolve once and move on. It hits different family members in different ways at different times. So we go through it often, if not continuously. We end up having to say, along with Dee, "I don't have any advice for you, because I don't even know what to do in my own situation."

We continue to talk about it, though, talk one another through it as it happens. Some of our conclusions: It's possible that our loved ones are scared witless of our illness. They resent our canes and crutches as symbols of their own helplessness and weakness even more than of our own frailties. They love us and want to protect us. But with MS, they're fighting an adversary that's so powerful and so sneaky that their attempts to defend us are futile. They end up feeling confounded, stymied in their efforts to support us. This makes them angry; perhaps the anger comes out as frustration with us rather than with our disease.

We remind ourselves and one another that there are stages of acceptance and understanding that relatives of people with chronic illness have to go through, just as we ourselves go through these stages. Sometimes our family members get stuck in the disbelief or denial stage. As long as we can get around on our own, they can say, "Well, she looks fine, so we can pretend she is fine." But add the cane into the mix, and suddenly we don't look so fine anymore. All of a sudden everybody is forced to face the fact that we need help walking, and there is nothing they, no matter how much they love us, can do about that.

▲▲▲

LORI — While I can trace symptoms and occurrences back to about age seventeen or eighteen, the majority of my MS-related problems showed up after my marriage to Steve. He has seen my strength and health deteriorate over the years. While he tries to be there for me as much as possible, he, too, has a hard time dealing with it because he can't do anything to "fix" it. He is very frightened that they still might find something that is terminal. His biggest fear in all of this is losing me. Ironically, the way he has chosen to "deal" with it is by pushing away from me. I think this is the reaction a lot of men have when in the same circumstances. Men are not raised to be able to deal with emotional issues such as these. They are taught to be the big, bad, macho males who have to take care of everything.

▲▲▲

DEE — Some members of my family kind of bug me, especially when I haven't seen them for a while. Maybe I'm limping, or I can't see very well at the moment. I am greeted with, "Now what's wrong?" I hate that. It's like I picked this illness and really enjoy having it attack different parts of my body!

One thing that has helped, though, is that a friend of mine has both multiple sclerosis and fibromyalgia; when she's around my husband or the rest of my family, she puts in little remarks about how hard it is to deal with the pain, fatigue, etc. I think her message is coming across, because tonight I rode the exercise bike for about five minutes, and when I told my husband, he said, "Be careful; you'll wear yourself out." You could have knocked me over with a feather! Do you have a friend nearby who could maybe drop the same kind of hints for your benefit?

If that doesn't work, just ignore others' comments. Nobody uses a cane just because it's fun.

▲▲▲

VICKI — I think there is a mask they hand you when you leave the neurologist's office after being diagnosed. I wear mine around my parents and most of the rest of family. I dreaded the first time my mom had to see me with the cane or in my wheelchair. She tried to hide her shock, but I could see it. I have no doubt she went home and cried for me. That kills me. I don't like anyone, especially my mom, to cry for me. I have heard that she once made a comment that she would rather I had had a baby out of wedlock than have MS. If you knew my mom, you would realize just how strong those words are.

▲▲▲

PAT — I met Bill (my husband) way before my diagnosis, though symptoms were surely present at the time. As far as dealing with MS, he is not always the greatest, though he does try. It is hard for him to understand that sometimes I can "appear" fine while falling apart inside. Yet when I needed crutches, or a wheelchair, or a hospital bed, or a porta-potty, or a wall-mounted mirror for my cathing expeditions, he was there helping me. And as time has gone by and he has seen that I can't always plan "outings," he has come to accept it a little better. I am not saying he likes it, but he does seem to accept it. He has stuck by me through more illnesses than most men would put up with. To me, that is God at work.

My kids have grown up only knowing "our mom is sick." It was simply a statement of fact in our house. In fact, two years in a row my son entered a grade-school essay contest, the subject being "Why My Mom Is A Supermom." In both essays, my MS was mentioned, though not by name. He simply said his mom was sick. And both times he won for his age and grade group. Needless to say, I was proud! My daughter was only about four years old when I was diagnosed, so to her a mom who was sick was just part of our lives. I never made a big deal out of it and they never did either. In this, I think God also played a major part in leading me.

▲▲▲

Sometimes we need to find a balance between denying that the MS's presence is a big deal and admitting that on some days, in some situations, its presence *is* a bigger deal than we can handle without our families' help.

▲▲▲

DONNA — I have heard each of us try to decide whether to tell our loved ones of our latest symptoms. We don't want to bother them, or we choose to wait until the time is more appropriate. As wives and mothers, we have learned to put aside our needs in favor of the needs of those we love. We make sacrifices in order to watch our families grow and prosper. No sacrifice is too great if our children or our spouses will benefit. We *love* our families and try to protect them. That is our job, our career, our life's work.

Then the MonSter or some other chronic and debilitating illness moves into our lives. We feel responsible for the changes our families will have to endure. We wonder if we will become a burden, emotionally, financially, or physically, on our loved ones. We tend to suffer in silence to avoid hearing ourselves whine or to avoid disruption for our families.

I think that sometimes we stay silent because 1) we don't want to be a burden; 2) we don't want to lose our independence; 3) that is our job, dammit; 4) we don't know how to let others be the caregivers; and 5) we are afraid of assuming less active roles in our families.

I am trying to look at this MeSs as an opportunity to grow. Before the MeSs moved in, I was the one doing and planning, predicting needs and meeting them ahead of time. An example I will use is the frequent family meals that include my husband, me, our three children and their spouses, and of course the grandbabies. Until a few months ago, I decided on the menu, did the shopping, prepared the food, served it, and then scatted the girls to the den or outside with the little ones while I cleaned up. Now we decide the menu by phone. Gary or one of the girls shops for whatever is needed. All of the girls come to my house, and the four of us do the cooking. Later, the girls clean up while I get to play with the grandbabies. I will admit that at first I had great difficulty relinquishing my kitchen and my job to the girls. MS changed our lives in this respect, but the rewards have been greater than the sacrifice.

If we become angry at the losses in our lives, we need to remember that the MonSter is the thief, and not wage war with those who love and cherish us. If we hide the things that are unpleasant from our loved ones in order to protect them, why should we be angry when their expectations of us remain too high?

I didn't intend to preach, and I hope that I have made sense and have not offended anyone. I think we need to let our families share all parts of our lives because, like it or not, until there is a cure, MS is here to stay. The ripples from the disease can make us or break us. I see my family as my life preservers. If I get helplessly caught up in the MS current, I want as many ropes around me as I can get.

▲▲▲

Jamie, in her poetic style, offers us hope that real love within a family can be its own protection against the effects of multiple sclerosis:

▲▲▲

This is a poem I wrote when I felt like my significant other was not accepting or understanding my fight with the MonSter. . . .

In words you say you love me
and accept me the way I am,
Sometimes actions speak much louder,
and I wonder if you even give a damn.
Fear and doubt creep through the cracks,
Permeate the windows of my soul,
Leaving within a chilling air
Obscuring sight of our real goal.
Then memories of all we've shared
come flooding back to mind—
The good, the bad, the laughter mixed—
a love with ties that bind.
Tears come and wash away
the pain within my heart.
Once again, I know for sure
our love did not depart. . . .
We claim progress, not perfection
and prove this every day,
When something is just meant to be,
True love will find the way. . . .

7

But You Look Too Good to Have MS!

We've seen that when our condition deteriorates to the point that we need help to get around, the sight of canes in our hands or crutches under our arms can have a profound, shocking impact on family members. This happens to some extent with people outside our families, too. Previously we might have been able to pass through any public place without attracting a second glance; we looked as "good" (normal? healthy?) as anybody else in the crowd. Then, the minute we use canes (or whatever) to help us walk, there's visual proof that we aren't so "good" after all. How many times have we passed a stroller in the grocery store aisle and heard its occupant say, "Mommy! What's the matter with that lady?"

Some people even zero in on precisely what is the matter. Five years ago, we were getting ready to move into a new house. I'd talked several times on the phone to Steve, the mover we'd hired. On the morning of the move, Steve rang our doorbell. I answered it and, leaning on my quad cane, showed him through the rooms that were to be emptied. After just a couple of minutes, he said, "You have MS, don't you?"

I was startled; had I mentioned that to him in our phone conversations? "What makes you say that?" I asked.

"My wife has it, too. It kind of shocked me when I saw you. You remind me of her—you're both good-looking ladies, if you don't mind me saying so. But as soon as I saw you walk, I knew what was wrong. You and she just kind of move the same way. She even has a cane exactly like that one!"

So there it was; the cane had eradicated somebody's first impression that I looked good! Even for people who are less astute than Steve or who had never paid attention to an MSer's walk, the cane screams, "Something is the matter with this lady!"

Although the disease is capable of affecting everything from the scalp to the toes, the focus of multiple sclerosis is on the legs. That's the first place people look for evidence when we tell them we have MS.

The ability or inability to walk is a major measuring stick in determining how "bad" the disease is in any individual. That's true even for official documentation of disability; it's only very recently that some of the accepted disability scales determine status based on more than just walking ability. The consensus has been that, if you have MS, you might be blind, deaf, unable to think clearly, unable to lift a fork to your lips, and unable to tend to your own personal needs. But if you can walk a hundred feet, then you're doing fine! Well, maybe it's not that cut and dried. But that's the general idea.

It's true that loss of feeling and/or function in the legs is one of the most common symptoms of MS. Maybe the legs are the easiest place for the MonSter to grab onto? I don't know—I'll leave that to the doctors to explain. But since most MSers eventually feel the effects of the disease in their legs, most of us ultimately face the need to use assistive devices in order to stay at least mobile, if not ambulatory.

It's hard when we arrive at that crossroads. It shouldn't be a big deal to start using a cane to add a bit of stability and balance to a walk or, if the time comes, to agree to sit down as we travel from one room to another. But in reality, having to use assistive devices means a lot more than just deciding to run to the medical supply store and pick out a cane. It means "giving in" to the disease, or at least acknowledging that the MonSter really is a viable entity in our lives. It means branding ourselves with labels like *crippled* or *disabled* or *handicapped* or *dependent*. It means making ourselves vulnerable to the curiosity of everyone who sees us. It means eating our words, words like, "I'll never get that bad. I'll never have to resort to that."

But resort we do, sooner or later. It was sooner for me. Once I got used to the idea that I had MS, and also to the idea that I could go for long periods of time with few or no symptoms, I didn't obsess over the thought that I might one day need help to get around. A couple of months after my diagnosis, I went to the hospital to visit a friend who'd fractured her spine. The parking garage at the hospital was being renovated, and I had to park several blocks away and walk uphill on a windy, icy day. I'd thought that since the MS was in remission I wouldn't have any problem. But a few steps into the excursion, my legs went back into their electric/tingling/numb/weak/useless mode. I had to sit down right then and there, on the sidewalk, and wait until I could move again. Then I practically crawled back to my car and just drove around the area until I found a closer parking place.

When I actually made it into the hospital my friend did *not* tell me that I looked too good to have MS. She looked at me, and then volunteered to get up out of the bed and let me take her place. Ron went out that evening and bought me my first cane.

So, it was an easy decision to make, right? Initially, yes, but it got shot down again pretty quickly. When I went for my next appointment with my neurologist, I thought about trying to walk from the parking lot to his office, decided I didn't want to spend the afternoon sitting on asphalt, and took the cane with me. As soon as Dr. M. saw it, he asked, "What are you doing with that thing? Did I tell you that you needed to use one of those?"

After that, it was hard for me to use the cane, even at times when I truly couldn't walk more than a few steps without it. I was afraid that I was being a hypochondriac, or that I was just looking for attention, or that my fear of falling meant that I was either neurotic or lazy.

In the following few years, I saw Dr. M. for several flare-ups of symptoms. Each time he said something like, "There's nothing wrong with you; you just have spring fever" or "You're just too introspective" or "You're like a bad penny; you just keep turning up." So I started to see a different neurologist, Dr. P., who confirmed the MS diagnosis and never mentioned canes or crutches or anything along those lines. At that point, I was trying to avoid using my cane whenever I could; I preferred to have Ron go with me everywhere, and especially to doctors' appointments. Most of the time I was fine, but when weakness or loss of balance appeared suddenly, I'd just lean on him for support. If I went shopping, even for one small item, I started out with a shopping cart right away so I'd have something to hang onto and keep me upright.

Then a change in our insurance forced me to switch neurologists again. That's when I met Dr. R., my present neurologist. During my first attack following the change, I went to see him, cane in hand. I apologized to his nurse as she led me to the examination room. "I try to do without the cane most of the time," I said, "but sometimes I just really need to use it."

"Don't you dare try to go without it!" she said. "We don't want to have to treat you for injuries from a fall on top of the MS."

A few minutes later, Dr. R. told me that he believes that his patients know more about their bodies than any doctor does, and that he basically expects them to let him know when they need treatment or any other assistance. Since that visit, I used the cane almost every waking minute, until I had to graduate to forearm crutches recently. I also use a wheelchair or electric scooter for long distances and on extra-bad days. I've never felt embarrassment, shame, or self-consciousness. I only feel a welcome security in having extra support when I need it, and more confidence in my own ability to discern how much added support I really need.

As we saw in the previous chapter, though, sometimes family

members or friends take over for us in the embarrassment, shame, or self-consciousness department.

▲▲▲

CHRIS — I had an interesting day yesterday! My husband and I went to an air show with his brother and his brother's wife. Well, I finally decided to use my cane! When my brother-in-law saw it, at first he didn't say anything, so I thought, "Okay, this is good!" Later in the day, he finally pointed to it and asked, "What is that for? *Sympathy?!*"

I said, "No, my doctor told me a month ago to start using it, but I expected reactions like yours, and that's exactly why I haven't used it until now." The subject was never brought up again. I guess this is to be expected, and it's just something else to get used to with this disease. I will survive!

▲▲▲

SHARON — Chris, here's what you do. You tell your brother-in-law that "Yes, the cane is for sympathy, and for this too!" Then you beat the living shit out of him with it. While he is in the hospital, you can give him all the freakin' sympathy he wants. And if you need help, I'm just a few hours away. I'll get the other Flutterbuds from this area, and we'll bring baseball bats and help you beat his sorry butt. (Okay, Sisters? I figure I can count on you for a good old Yankee beating of a jerk.)

▲▲▲

Some MSers hold out until the decision can't be postponed any longer.

▲▲▲

BARB — Well, gang, I know I shouldn't complain, because I'm not in bad shape for the shape I'm in. But the stumbling and bumbling have now resulted in a big-time fall. I was leaving the office, made it down nine steps from the office suite to the main door, where there are two more steps to the parking lot.

I just couldn't navigate those two steps. I don't know if I lost my balance or if my blurry vision made me misstep or what. I fell right on my face onto the asphalt parking lot. I scraped my knee and tore a big hole in my slacks. A man across the parking lot asked, "Hey, are you okay?" I answered, "Sure, I'm just trying out a new trick." So he went on, while I sat there trying to figure out how to get up.

I ended up with just a lovely bruise and one small cut, so it's nothing awful. But then. . . .

This made me wonder. Was this a definite use-a-cane-before-you-really-get-hurt warning, or just one of those things that can happen to anybody? I hate to make too much of it, but I am trying to learn when to adapt, as we're always talking about. Please give me your input. Am I stupid or what?

▲▲▲

DONNA — I had several close calls before I decided to check out some canes (actually, the neurologist told me to quit being stubborn and get a cane before I broke my fool neck). It felt very awkward at first. I felt I was drawing attention to myself and my inability to walk a straight line. So the cane stayed in my car for the first few days. I would look at it and decide to leave it there while I walked like a drunken woman into the stores.

When I finally worked up the courage to use the cane, I found I could walk for longer periods without tiring. I didn't realize how hard I had been working just to keep my balance. At first I felt very conspicuous and felt I had given in to the MS. But now I see that using a cane is actually a way to take back some control.

In the time b.c. (before cane), some mothers would frown at me as they ushered their children out of my stumbling path, and others would just give me this questioning look. Now, since the cane, it's nice to see smiles again.

I now have several canes. I keep one by each of the exterior doors to our house and one in each of our vehicles. I don't use one inside the house except on very bad days or when I'm really tired and tip over easily.

I'd recommend that you go for it. Try several canes, and pick the one(s) that feel comfortable to you.

▲▲▲

DEE — Barb, I'm sorry about your fall but glad you weren't hurt too badly. I've been struggling with the same issue: whether or not it's time to get a cane. Some days I do fine, but there are days when I just bounce from one wall to the other, blah blah blah, you know how that story goes. I had that same kind of fall, going into the drugstore. The people who happened to be there were very kind. They just gathered around and helped me up (embarrassing, but appreciated). I ripped a hole in the knee of my favorite jeans, but as far as getting hurt, I only skinned my knees and one ankle.

I still haven't gotten a cane. But I've been thinking about it. This idea of using assistive devices is a difficult issue. Yet when I see people using canes or whatever they need to get around, I don't think anything of it. I don't even pay that much attention, unless I see that they need assistance.

▲▲▲

JAMIE — Barb, dear, I'm very sorry you fell. Here's my input: I navigate in the house without my cane or crutch (by wall-walking, chair-grabbing, etc.). But after many, many falls, I put my pride on the back burner and stopped trying to be "normal" when walking outside. I still go out sometimes without my leg brace, but not without my cane.

It's no shame to use a cane. The shame is in needing one

and refusing to use it. Be safe, Barb, and be good to yourself. Use the cane!

▲▲▲

We've found benefits to using canes (or other aids) that extend beyond the added safety:

1. Using an assistive device elicits curiosity from onlookers, but that's better than fear or unsolicited judgments as to your state of inebriation.

2. Store security personnel stop following you around so closely, as they no longer assume that you've drunkenly wandered into their store by mistake.

3. People are pleased to hold doors open, give up their places in line, pick up dropped items, and offer whatever assistance they can when they see that you have a legitimate need for help.

4. If the cane is three- or four-footed and can stand on its own, it provides a handy hanger for purse, shopping bag, or hat when you sit down.

▲▲▲

TARA — Barb, I hope that you're not hurt too badly. We've probably all done that stunt once or twice, too. Heal quickly, and say yes to the cane. If nothing else, it lets people know to give you a bit more room, and it alerts them that "there is more to this fall than sheer clumsiness." I've also found that using a cane helps to let people know other things, too:

1. Yes, it would be nice if you would hold that door open for me.

2. No, please do not honk for me to cross this parking lot (street, whatever) any faster than I am.

3. Please keep those little ankle biters away from me while I try to maneuver.

4. Yes, I would like some help to get the groceries to the car.

5. *Yes, I do belong in this handicapped parking space!*

▲▲▲

Which brings up two more often-mentioned topics among MSers: How do you deal with the looks you get when you use your state-sanctioned handicapped placard and then get out of the car and appear to walk normally across the parking lot? And how do you deal with the person who doesn't have a handicapped placard but parked in the last handicapped spot anyway, and then got out of the car and walked normally across the parking lot?

▲▲▲

LORI — Sometimes when I'm walking around with my cane and/or choose to use my handicapped placard on bad days, I get a lot of weird looks (I'm only twenty-eight and look younger, or so people say). At those times, I'd love to have a sign that says, "I have MS, so what's your problem?"

I'm sure most people think I'm some sort of insurance fraud person or something of the kind. People my age aren't supposed to need canes and handicapped parking spots. After all, I just "look so good!"

▲▲▲

Helen lives in a large city in the Midwest. She tells us:

▲▲▲

This seems to be party city for illegal parkers. Go to any grocery store and who is in the handicapped parking? Young guys with loud boom boxes and an attitude. Since I don't want to get shot and add to the crap I already deal with, I try to find a security guard. Some of them will make the parkers move; some look at you like you're nuts for asking them to do their job.

One day I was having a very bad time, and as I pulled into my parking place, this old man came walking up and asked me why I was parking there, since I obviously wasn't disabled. I looked him square in the eye, pulled myself up to my full five feet two inches, and said, in a very businesslike tone, "I'm legally blind and a crazed ax murderer. Any further questions?" Then I just walked away. I hope he didn't have a heart attack!

Then there was the time I went to park at Best Buy and some twenty-something woman beat me to the last handicapped spot. I was actually polite and simply asked, "Do you know that this is disabled parking?" To which she responding by asking if it was any of my fucking business. When I explained to her that I have license plates with a disabled emblem, she said, "Fuck you, bitch, you don't look very disabled to me. I'm parking here." I went to the store manager that time.

So as someone who has had it with both barrels from both sides, I can empathize with what happens to all of you. I try to be polite, but I'm not afraid to ask, "Are you aware that this is handicapped parking?" That usually does the trick; it's non-confrontational, and few people get mad.

▲▲▲

Most of us will admit that when we see an apparently healthy person get out of a car with no tag in a handicapped slot, our first assumption is "Schmuck!" But we realize that there are many disabilities that do not display themselves by abnormal gait or crutches or wheelchairs, and many reasons one may not have a placard on the car. So when we see the pretty young thing jump out of her sporty little tagless car and go bopping off to her aerobics class, we do try to be compassionate or at least diplomatic if we point out her mistake.

That's a safety measure, too. We've all heard the news stories, so we try to remember that if we jump out and start yelling at someone, even that pretty young thing, she's liable to pull a gun on us! She isn't likely to say, "Oh, wait, I can't shoot this person; she has a handicapped placard!"

I occasionally run (ha!) into times when somebody sees me with a cane and concludes that my only disability is my advanced age. The first time this happened I was in my early thirties, thank you very much! I was taking my dogs for a walk up and down our street, using my quad cane for support. I passed a little boy, one of our new next-door neighbors, sitting on his front steps. He wanted to see the dogs, so I invited him to come out and pet them. After he did, he ran back into his house yelling, "Mama, Mama! I petted that puppy!"

"Whose puppy did you pet?" I heard Mama ask.

He answered, "That old lady that lives next door."

I waited for somebody to tell me, "But you look too good to be old!" Nobody did.

▲▲▲

PAT — Because I've already been through living in a wheelchair and/or using crutches, I thought I'd offer my thoughts on this topic. We've talked about being unable to do as much as you once did, passing up invitations and not going to places you once loved to visit, backing off from doing certain things that once brought you pleasure. There's one question that I have come to rely on when deciding whether to take my wheelchair or both crutches, or even get by with one crutch: Will using something allow me to do this activity?

I wound up in a wheelchair suddenly, so my first agenda was to get *out* of that dang thing. I graduated to crutches and then went back to work with no walking aids at all. But some good things don't last, and I found myself struggling to get around. In order to keep working, I gave in and used one crutch, figuring this wasn't as bad as a wheelchair. I pushed myself constantly, doing whatever I could and paying for it later with severe pain and spasms. Before long, I had to leave my job. I was down to doing only one or two things a week, backing away from family and friends' invitations, turning down my husband's suggestions for dinner out, a movie, or just a car ride for ice cream.

Calls from friends asking me to go places became less frequent. After all, I did say, "No thanks" more than "I'd love to." My family, who disliked my using a wheelchair more than I care to admit, started to suggest I take it along "just in case." The signs that I was overdoing it were there, but it took me a while to see them for myself. And once I did see them, it took longer to figure out how to deal with this unwanted situation. Once I found I was living my life more by myself than with family and friends, the loneliness set in. And with it came the realization that I was being a complete idiot!

That's when I discovered that using crutches or a wheelchair or a handicapped card on my windshield could actually mean freedom for me. Slowly, I began the task of finding what was "okay" for me. If I was going on a quick trip to the store, the crutches would be fine. For a trip to the mall, the wheelchair would let me stay longer, and spend more money! Yes, there were problems with going in the wheelchair (e.g., getting help opening the ladies' room door, getting around aisles in the crowded stores, having to skip some stores because they were too small to accommodate a wheelchair, not to mention carrying the packages). But the pros far outweighed the cons.

It wasn't easy to find a balance at first, and I still struggle with it now. However, I do know my limitations to a better degree, and I no longer have to turn down invitations unless I truly feel I'm not up to it. When I am invited to do something, I only decline if I don't want to or don't feel well, not because I may need to use some assistance. Doing things in this way helps me to use my muscles when I am able and give them a break when I know they can't take the stress. Fatigue is kept to a minimum.

I must admit that there are times when I'm having a good day and feel like I can sneak by, doing more than I should. And I do pay for that: if not the next day, then within the next few days. Something will *always* start to bother me, be it fatigue, muscle weakness, a leg that "forgets" to move when I'm walking, an arm that's too weak to lift a pencil, or that bandlike sensation around my chest.

Learning when something is too much or not enough is an individual experience. I don't believe there is a set answer that fits us all. The decision to get walking aids or special parking favors comes when you see life passing you by and you still want to participate. There's a happy medium for each person. The challenge is to find what's most important to you and what works best for you, and take it from there. It's not an easy challenge, but it is one that can be dealt with.

▲▲▲

Thanks, Pat. I guess that what it all boils down to is that other people's impressions of us as MSers are inconsequential. If I go somewhere in a wheelchair, probably about half of the people who see me, if they bother to react or even to notice me at all, will assume that I'm lazy, that I'm trying to get attention, or that I'm seeking special treatment. The other half will likely wonder briefly what happened to me and then dismiss their own curiosity as unimportant. Which is exactly what it is. What *is* important is my own acceptance of the fact that, if I hope to get on with my life in the fullest possible sense, I'll have to rely on something besides "looking good" to get me where I want to go.

8

Yes, It Hurts

JANE

Pain

That inhumane visitor
Came again last night
That cruel master of the mind
Subverter of peace
Enemy of the soul
Perverted passion personified
Searing seductress of sanity
The pain which threatens Life
Limits reality and usurps
Every joy and worthwhile moment
Intrusive and destructive
My body screams for it to leave
But nothing helps

I have to admit that if I'd read this poem seven or eight years ago, I would have thought, "Gee, Jane must have something wrong besides MS. Multiple sclerosis could never cause that much pain."

I admit further that I was just plain naive back then. I used to think that pain was, and forever would be, the least of my worries about multiple sclerosis. MS wasn't a particularly painful condition, right? That's what all the doctors and medical books said back then. Pain was for those unfortunate people who had cancer or rheumatism; it wasn't something that I had to be anxious about.

The biggest concerns for me, during the initiation/education phase of this disease, were numbness and weakness. At the time of my diagnosis, I'd lost feeling and mobility in my legs and, a few months later, in my left arm and hand. At that time, I would have welcomed pain, would have been thrilled to be able to feel the I.V. needle being inserted into my forearm during my daily steroid treatments. I would have jumped at the chance to stub my toe and feel the soreness vibrate up to my knee. (I would have jumped at the chance to jump at anything!) Pain was, in my mind, a feeling, a sure sign that life was still present somewhere in my useless limbs. And where there was life, I theorized, there was hope for recovery. During those early days of relapse/remission, I did eventually recover, at least to some extent, every time the MS attacked. Each exacerbation left me more determined to remain strong enough to ward off future attacks.

With that in mind, I began to walk every chance I got. During my lunch breaks at work, I'd travel all the Cincinnati streets within a five-block circumference of my downtown office building. Then, after work, I'd go home, put my dogs on their leashes, and head out again. I grew addicted to, almost obsessed with, walking. When I walked, I felt physically energized, mentally alert, emotionally relaxed, spiritually refreshed. Multiple sclerosis, especially pain associated with multiple sclerosis, was the farthest thing from my mind. I was in control of what happened to my body. When little tingles or bouts of "sleepiness" did show up in my legs or arms, I was able to ignore them and keep right on with my walking regime.

I even won second place in a walking contest, initiated by the editor of the newspaper I worked for to encourage his employees to stay fit. The $35 prize was a nice bonus, but nothing compared to the supreme satisfaction I found in having outdistanced the Mon-Ster, at least for a while.

At about that time, reports began to surface that said that pain should indeed be recognized as a primary effect of multiple sclerosis. Several of the doctors I saw at the time asked me at every visit if I was having trouble with pain. I assured them that I had no pain then and wouldn't in the future. Walking was to be my salvation, I was certain. As long as I kept my legs strong and in motion, pain, numbness, and all the other MS muck couldn't catch up with me. I could just walk away from it.

I marvel now at my credulity. All too soon, I found out that my self-righteous pride in staying as ambulatory as possible was no defense against the raw hurt that overtook me. Despite all my scoffing at pain over the years, I soon was, and am now, being fed a steady diet of my own words. When I head out with my dogs for our walks now, I have to arm myself with crutches, muscle relaxers, and painkillers, along with prayers that I'll be able to cover the length of six or seven houses before the pain (combined with numbness and fatigue) sends me back home. More often than not, before I've gone past even three houses, my legs and hips go completely spastic. Each step makes them feel like they're being pulled in opposite directions, that they're connected to the rest of my body only by the agonizing ache that starts in my arches and extends up to my midsection. Sometimes I push myself to keep on, and arrive home close to tears. Other times I exercise some sense and turn around as soon as the spasms start.

I miss the days when I could take off and just keep going until one of the dogs got tired; that always happened long before I felt any fatigue or pain. I still can't let go of my love for walking. Nor can I give up the idea that my pain would be much worse if I didn't walk as much as possible. But since my "as much as possible" desire to walk is tied more and more to an "as little as possible" pain endurance level, I've at last learned to modify my efforts.

I wish I could say that my legs are the only area affected by pain. No such luck. Over the past few years, I've come up with (down with?) almost constant pain in my neck and shoulders, all the way down my spine, through my arms down to the hands, and, at times, surrounding my entire rib cage. (I've heard others refer to that last discomfort as the "MS hug." Some hug!) Sometimes I wake during the night feeling as if a steel rod has been jammed through each of my bones.

Is it all due to MS? I don't know. I've been diagnosed at various times with systemic lupus erythematosis, rheumatoid arthritis, polyarthritis, and fibromyalgia. Almost all the MSers I know have at least one of these painful conditions in addition to MS. So it's hard to sort out. But there is progress, because now medical professionals really recognize pain as a bona fide manifestation of multiple sclerosis.

▲▲▲

JOY — I just read that there is now evidence that MS is not painless, as used to be the common belief. While the majority of people with multiple sclerosis don't have pain as a predominant symptom, about 80 percent of people with MS experience related pain at least occasionally. And an estimated 5 to 15 percent of those with the disease have chronic pain.

Well, I happen to think too many in our Froup experience pain, whether the cause is multiple sclerosis or fibromyalgia or something else. *I'm tired of it!* I'm going to have a serious talk with somebody important and powerful about just making it go away!

(But I'll try to be diplomatic about it, because the Somebody is pretty High Up.)

▲▲▲

We can certainly assume that much of our pain, no matter how many companion conditions we each have, is at least peripherally connected to MS. MS, for one thing, causes muscle spasms, which can be very painful. It can cause a lopsided, unbalanced gait and posture, which can strain muscles and exert excess pressure on bones and soft tissues.

What's more, multiple sclerosis can distort sensory messages to and from the brain, so that the stroke of a feather ends up being about as tolerable as a smack with a baseball bat. It can inflame the nerves in any area of the body that it decides to invade, causing violent pain in that region.

Not long ago, Renee was hit with agonizing face pain. This was new to her; she didn't know at first whether it was caused by a bad tooth, an eye problem, a sinus infection, thrush, or something else.

▲▲▲

I never knew that pain could be so painful! This beats everything else that has ever hurt me. My teeth hurt, my jaw hurts, my eyes hurt, even my tongue hurts so bad I can't eat. I can't write any more about it right now, because I took some pain pills and now have to go lie down.

I have an appointment coming up with my neurologist. Meanwhile, does anybody have any idea of what's going on here?

▲▲▲

TARA — Renee, recently I went to my dentist because of that same kind of pain. He found no sinus issues, no cavities, no nothing. His assessment was that it is the MS affecting one of the nerves. It is really impossible to tell for sure until they get in there and x-ray the whole thing.

I know that the pain is horrid, and I think that at some point the doctors may consider severing the nerve. But since I'm not a doctor, I'm not sure. I am glad that you are going to a specialist. I hope he will be able to answer some of the questions around this and relieve the pain somehow.

▲▲▲

SALLY — I had this pain (it's called trigeminal neuralgia) sooooooo bad that I almost killed myself with a combination of analgesics, none of which, by the way, touched the pain. I had been to the dentist (no help) and a neurologist (no help). It was so horrid that sometimes I lay on my floor moaning. One night I just couldn't stand it anymore and went to the emergency room.

At the first one I went to, the doctor brushed me off as if it was nothing and told me to see a dentist. Then he charged me extra for "misusing the ER." I was in such pain that I just stayed in my truck and cried because I couldn't drive. After it eased up a bit, I started to go home and it hit again. I went to a different ER, and they took me seriously. They asked me to smell something in a little bottle and tell them what it smelled like (don't ask me why), and then they came back in and gave me a shot of something. They asked if I had a way home, because I wouldn't be able to drive after a few minutes. I told them I had my truck in the parking lot and could sleep in my camper if they would okay it with the security guard, which they did. Boy, were they right! The shot knocked me out, but it killed the pain. I hadn't had *any* sleep for three days before that and it was such a relief. After that, if I took strong pain relievers when the pain first started, it would stop it before it got so bad.

▲▲▲

RENEE [Later] — I went to the doctor today (my neurologist), and guess what: This is yet another nerve-pain symptom of MS. It hurts like hell, especially my tongue. The doctor took one look and said, "Yes—this is definitely MS pain."

Oh, wonderful. Not only does it hurt to eat or drink, it hurts like shit to *not* eat or drink. Plus nothing has any taste. The doctor says it should go away soon. Yeah, right.

▲▲▲

Within the next few days, Renee's trigeminal neuralgia joined forces with an attack of optic neuritis, causing excruciating eye pain. At that point, she agreed to her doctor's suggestion that she have a series of intravenous steroid treatments. She ultimately was able to get some relief (temporarily) through these treatments.

Part of our pain-management dilemma is that some doctors are reluctant to prescribe narcotic pain relievers, especially when pain is chronic or recurring. In some ways, this is understandable, because of the potential for abuse. On the other hand, it's commonly understood that those patients who really need strong, long-term medication for pain control are the least likely to abuse the drugs or become dependent on them beyond pain relief. Worse, some doctors won't even prescribe nonnarcotic analgesics that for one reason or another don't fit their own criteria of "acceptable" drugs.

I've had my own (un)memorable experience with this recently. The rheumatologist I'd seen years ago for treatment of lupus/fibromyalgia/whatever-it-is had no problem with prescribing whatever was needed for pain relief. In fact, I think he was too generous in this respect. I'm sure that at that point I could have managed with ibuprofen most of the time. But this doctor insisted that part of long-term management involved staying ahead of the pain, which was more effectively accomplished with a combination of ibuprofen and prescription painkillers. So I took both, with no trouble. I don't think I came even close to being dependent on the drugs, although I did get kind of addicted to being pain-free for a few hours a day. But I didn't really like this particular doctor, and I decided after a couple of years to quit seeing him. My primary-care doctor, Dr. C., okayed that decision, but he told me that he "would not" prescribe narcotics. That was fine with me. I'd manage, I was sure.

More recently, though, the discomfort increased to the point at which I began to wake at night in tears; I wasn't able to sleep more than a few hours at a time. So I asked Dr. C. about a particular nonsteroidal/nonnarcotic analgesic (Ultram), which many of the Flutterbuds had recommended as very effective against this particular type of pain. He told me that he "just won't use it." I wanted to say, "I'm not asking you to use it; I'm just asking you to prescribe it," but as usual, I wimped out and muttered my usual nonconfrontational bow-down-to-the-doctor reply: "Oh, okay."

He told me to instead take 400 milligrams of ibuprofen every four hours. I almost laughed, since I'd been living more on ibuprofen than on food for the past six months. Then, as I was checking out at the appointment desk, he came out of an exam room and said, "You're right, the ibuprofen won't be enough for your kind of pain." Then he wrote a prescription for another nonsteroidal/nonnarcotic, which I'd used before and had found even less effective than ibuprofen. Nevertheless, I was willing to try it again. That is, until he said, "You can take this twice a day" and handed me a prescription for twenty pills! Well, no thank you, Dr. C.! I'm not going to make a thirty-day insurance copayment on a ten-day supply of pills that have so far done zilch for pain relief.

I went home feeling that Dr. C. hadn't paid a bit of attention to anything I'd said. It was as if his hearing shut down as soon as I mentioned using a drug that wasn't in his particular pharmacopoeia. I went home and gave myself a few days to "cool down" and try to find ways to cope. But each night, as the painful pressure of my own body against the bed sent me to the sofa to sleep sitting up, and each day, as I megadosed on ibuprofen, my anger and frustration reignited.

After a few days, I wrote a letter to Dr. C. I began by explaining that I'd chosen to write because I have so much trouble communicating on the phone and because I didn't care to go through the details of my problem with his receptionist. I told him again the extent of the pain that I was dealing with and detailed the ways in which it seemed to adversely affect every area of my life. I listed the reasons why I didn't want to change doctors: I'd been more than satisfied with his care up to that point; I'd felt that a good doctor/patient relationship had grown between us over the seven years I'd been seeing him; I appreciated the convenient location of his office (very close to my house), since it would be a hardship to get transportation to another area. I closed with a plea for help, mailed the letter, and waited three weeks for an answer.

The "answer" was a phone call from his receptionist, telling me that Dr. C. had arranged for me to see the staff at a pain-control center thirty miles from my house! I said, "No thanks," told her to cancel my next appointment, and made an appointment with a friend's much-liked primary-care physician whose office is just a bit farther than Dr. C.'s office from my house.

My new primary-care doctor, Dr. B. (is anybody keeping track? Have I made it through the alphabet yet?), is much more generous with time, undivided attention, and prescriptions for needed pain remedies. That translates to me as much more caring about the real needs of his patients. From now on, I won't continue to see a doctor who doesn't demonstrate this same concern. If that ever happens again, though, I will do one thing differently. I'll confront my doctor immediately, while my anger is strongest. I'll take as much time as I need, and I won't budge from his/her office until I've managed to mumble and stumble my way through my speech. I won't do him/her the honor of a diplomatic, thought-out letter. And if I don't get the care I need, I won't bother to make another appointment.

Jane recently sent a letter to a friend of hers who was working closely with the National Multiple Sclerosis Society on the pain-control issue. It pretty much expresses the feelings of the rest of us, too.

▲▲▲

Dear Kay,

I welcome this opportunity to be heard by the National Multiple Sclerosis Society on pain. Thank you for alerting us.

I have had an MS diagnosis (probable) since 1973, confirmed by a positive MRI in 1988. I have spent much of this time in one kind of pain or another, although I have and have had only benign (slight) MS.

My physical pain was unrecognized by the medical community for many, many years—and for psychic self-preservation, I finally stopped talking about it. I actually stopped going to doctors for the most part. I coped by myself and went on with my life despite several kinds of pain and many kinds of obnoxious, squirrelly feelings and weird symptoms. I finally had my sanity confirmed when I read all about the things I'd been experiencing (for twenty-plus years) on [the Internet] about a year and a half ago.

Because I was not a participating, learning person with MS, I had missed the advances in medicine since my diagnosis. At the beginning, I was advised not to dwell on the diagnosis and told that there was only one medication (ACTH) that they could use, and I was to "save that for the big stuff"—which, thankfully, never came.

Just this past year, I have acquired a new neurologist who has put me on a number of medicines that have helped me a great deal. It took me using the word "torture" to get these from my good doctor. It quite naturally blew my mind to have instant relief! It's hard not to be bitter about all those "wasted" years! The pain was what I'd call of medium intensity. But the unrelenting nature of it made it absolutely maddening! I honestly thought there was no nonnarcotic medicine available to give me, since it was totally beyond my ken that if help existed, some doctor I'd seen would not have given it to me!

Even with the very best spiritual and mental discipline and training, pain is the absolute pits! It is dehumanizing and invades every aspect of a person's life.

Debilitating pain is just that—debilitating! Whether the spasms cause the muscle soreness or the pain comes from damaged nerves doesn't really concern me. I have MS and I have a great deal of pain! It is sheer folly for someone to say MS does not cause pain. I am a facilitator of two MS online chats and I attend another weekly one, and I can guarantee that many, many MS patients have a significant amount of pain! The estimate of how many patients do have pain (5 to 15 percent) sounds conservative to me. [N.B.: Jane was right. Studies conducted after Jane wrote this letter conclude that 55 percent of MSers have "clinically significant pain," meaning that a physician is able to assess the pain or observe its effects. Chronic pain affects nearly half (48 percent) of MS patients.] If you're one of the ones who have chronic pain, numbers don't matter anyway. I frequently spend much of my day either running from the pain (staying super busy) or begging family members for muscle rubs to try to eliminate it.

And then there's the whole area of jaw/neck/ear/cheek/head pain! For many years, I've had sudden stabbing pain as well as "sore to beat the band"-type pains. I often sit without motion when a wave comes on me, simply enduring it until it is over. It can be triggered, it seems, by a cold breeze, or by nothing at all. There is no real rhyme or reason to this pain, and it is maddening! I also endure those lightning spears in the eyes sometimes, or even intense pain in one finger! My body is always surprising me. Even after all these years, I feel new things almost weekly.

While I am not personally quite ready for narcotics, I greatly empathize with the many people who are. There damned well better be a place for me to turn to if and when I get to that point. Anything else is absolutely criminal and inhumane! And I can guarantee that I will find the one person who will give me access to the medication I need to live life relatively painlessly. I owe that to myself and to the God who made me, as well as to the family I love.

Just as there are doctors who are pitifully slow to join the merciful ones who don't worry about addiction in terminal illnesses, there are, I hope, an ever-increasing number of patients who refuse to settle for less than humane treatment. How sad that we, as a country, spend billions of dollars on any number of other things, yet allow some people to suffer from treatable pain. When will we ever learn?

Sincerely, Jane E. D.

▲▲▲

And I wonder when doctors will learn that the energy a patient expends trying to fight pain, or even to endure it, could be more effectively used to recover from an illness or injury?

Jane makes a very good point toward the end of her letter. If enough patients are unwilling to settle for less than humane care, maybe doctors will be forced to change their methods of caring. Patients with multiple sclerosis would, I think, be good ones to set this change in motion. Pain is one thing that all of us with multiple sclerosis share. Each of us, sooner or later, will experience pain that just doesn't want to quit.

Yes, MS hurts. Sometimes it hurts like hell.

9

Thank You, Mr. Fleet ... and Other Bathroom Stuff

VICKI — What is it with peeing?

Damn, I bought the super-duper styrofoam-lined incontinence pads. I have wasted (as in "didn't need them after all") damn near $16 worth of pads. I had myself convinced I could do without them. I've done exactly that for quite a while now. Then today I went into a convenience store to get supplies for Zach's [Vicki's son] lunch, and immediately I could feel it coming.

It was too late to find a john; besides, I'd given the clerk my money and wanted my change. Luckily, I didn't leak a lot, but any is more than I care to do in a public place. I managed to get into the van, sat on a brand new *People* magazine (gotta protect the upholstery!), and made it home with only one other small accident. As I walked in the door, Larry met me with, "I'm glad you're home, etc., etc. ...." I pushed past and explained that I was currently peeing in my pants and would talk to him after I showered.

One would think that, after a while, we would stop this shit and be able to act our age and not like a one-year-old.

Dammit, I'll be forty years old in a little while, and I would rather not be in diapers when I get there!

I'm finished. I think. I'm going to bed now.

▲▲▲

ME — Aww, Vicki, I know just what you mean!

▲▲▲

I'm sure that after her letter came through our E-mailboxes, Vicki's E-mailbox was subsequently flooded (oops! Sorry, Vicki! No pun intended!) with responses exactly like mine. We all do know the humiliation that Vicki experienced that day.

The fear of that humiliation governs every move that takes us away from the sanctity of our own bathrooms. It doesn't matter that we're only going to the post office for a book of stamps or the corner store for a quart of milk. We'd better know ahead of time the location of the restroom in the post office or the store. If an establishment doesn't have a public restroom or even a semipublic one (as in, "Please, sir, if you'll give me the key for just five minutes, I'll give you all my business for the next year!"), we'll probably just not go there.

When one of us summons enough courage to plan a long car trip (for some, "long" might translate to "more than ten miles away"; but we'll completely suspend disbelief and imagine, maybe, a hundred miles), the others in the Froup don't bother extending wishes for safe travel, good weather, reasonable hotel rates, or exciting experiences. It's enough to say, "May you find a rest area right away whenever you need one." That is the ultimate good wish, the most necessary blessing.

I don't know of a single MSer who doesn't have at least occasional problems with bladder and bowel control. It's easy to understand the problem, at least in theory; bowel and bladder control is dependent on the transmission of a message from the brain to the nether regions, telling the organs there to store bodily wastes for a reasonable length of time and then to eliminate those wastes more or less on command. With MS, the elimination happens sooner or later, but it occurs less as a response to a conscious command by the eliminator and more as a response to the body's own whims.

Sometimes lack of control is related to an episode of numbness in the pelvic or abdominal area. In that case, the person may not be aware that the bladder or bowels are in need of emptying. Sensory perception might be so muffled or distorted that there's no recognizable warning of impending overfill or overflow.

On the other hand, "MSers"/"people with MS" may experience urinary frequency or urgency, even at times when there shouldn't be any urgent need to urinate, e.g., immediately after the bladder has been emptied or when liquids have been eschewed to the point of dehydration. It doesn't matter—the brain of a person with MS can, at the slightest provocation, send a mixed-up signal, screaming that the bladder is full.

Since our sensory perception is less than trustworthy, it's hard to tell whether the feeling of urgency is a real warning or a false alarm. Inevitably, if the signal is ignored, it turns out to have been a real warning. Eventually, some little internal switch connected to the bladder gets flipped, the bladder empties of its own accord, and the MSer slinks off in total humiliation.

On the other hand, rushing to heed the alarm right away often results in a kind of internal freeze that, in spite of squeezings and pushings and prayers, won't allow even a drop to escape.

A number of years ago, I seemed to be in total remission. I had no trouble at all walking or coordinating my movements. I had no idea that bladder problems due to multiple sclerosis could be present even during an otherwise quiet phase. Evidently I underestimated the powers of the MonSter.

I was spending three weeks in Europe with Ron, the girls, and my sister Joyce and her husband, Herm. We spent most of our time visiting or traveling with one or more priests. That in itself made any kind of "private" problem even more embarrassing. A lot of the time, we were in areas where restroom facilities were few and far between. That meant that every time I did see a ladies' room, I took advantage of it. And, of course, I ran into the "not able to go" problem.

There must have been a couple of dozen times during those weeks when I'd go into a public restroom, thinking I could stay ahead of the game. Then I'd get stuck there, waiting for results, long past the time when the rest of the party was ready to move on. Making things still worse was the fact that in most public places in Italy at that time, the toilet was simply a drain in the concrete floor, with a little ledge on either side on which to stand. Not very conducive to ease in emptying the bladder! I'd usually end up unable to go at all. Then ten minutes later, I'd get a real warning, the kind not to be ignored. At that point, I'd have to ask our current clerical host to find the next available stop ASAP, and then I'd pray that he could accommodate my needs. Fortunately, I still had some modicum of control at the time, so I didn't have to suffer through anything worse than a few (very) close calls.

For that I thank God, especially when I hear stories like the one Renee tells us:

▲▲▲

Two years ago Burt and I went out west to participate in a Jeep Jamboree, where we'd get groups of twelve Jeeps in a line and drive on these ridiculously narrow mountain roads, 'round and 'round, without an inch to spare, in the freezing cold. Then we'd stop at an old mining town for a catered lunch. Actually, it was fun. Except when you had to use the bathroom, because there weren't any. At one of our roadside stops, I had to go, *now*, no matter that there wasn't a building with a restroom anywhere in sight.

So off I went up this steep hill to sit on a very cold rock (and I do mean cold) to pee. Of course, trying to pee is a major effort for me anyway, including lots of grunts and straining and, most probably, strange facial expressions, especially if I don't have the sound of running water to help me get going.

Anyway, there I sat with my pants down around my knees, trying to hold myself up with both hands to keep from sitting directly on this cold rock, just grunting and doing all the associated carrying-on. Two feet to the left of me, along came a man wearing a backpack, carrying a walking stick, and whistling. He proceeded to walk up to me, said good morning, stopped like he wanted to chat. At that point, I had actually started peeing, and once I start I can't turn it off. So there I semi-sat, peeing, talking to this hiker like it was the most natural thing in the world. Well, I peed in the wrong direction, which meant that in order to pull my pants up I had to first sit back down and reposition myself, and the only place to do so was on the cold, and now wet, rock. Since I have no sense of balance, I had no choice but to ask this man to pull me up and hold onto me so I could reach down and pull up my pants. He continued chatting about birds, nature, what have you. When I finished and said thanks, he said, "No problem!" and merrily went about his way, whistling on down the trail, never looking back.

Is life strange or what? I went back down the hill and told Burt what had happened. He, of course, told the rest of the group that night at dinner. They thought it was a hoot!

That was the last Jeep Jamboree I went on. However, since I am now the proud owner of a potty seat that sets up anywhere (it looks just like a baby potty seat, only it's grown-up size), I am ready to take on the world.

▲▲▲

I wish I had known before my trip to Europe that there are medications and procedures available that are very helpful in dealing with the "P-problem." My present neurologist eventually put me on oxbutynin, a drug specifically for urinary incontinence associated with conditions such as MS. I now take it whenever I know that I'll be away from a restroom for any length of time. It usually relieves the bladder spasticity enough that I can last through two or three hours with no worries about incontinence. It's been a real lifesaver for me.

Even before I started the drug, though, the wonderful internist I was seeing at the time arranged for a nurse to come to my house and teach me how to self-catheterize. I didn't think I was ready for or in need of such drastic measures. I wasn't planning any more trips to Europe in the near future, and I figured I could handle just about anything that happened if I stayed in familiar surroundings. Besides, I dreaded going through the learning process, which I imagined had to be utterly humiliating.

I'm grateful now that I let Dr. S. talk me into it. The nurse who showed up was sweet, upbeat, and very matter-of-fact in her approach. She had me sit on the edge of the bed, facing the wall mirror and holding a cup to catch the urine. Then she showed me how to prepare the area with an antiseptic swab and, wearing sterile rubber gloves, to lubricate the catheter and insert it into the urethra to drain the bladder. Keeping track of all the steps involved was much harder than the actual cathing.

I've since learned from a urologist that I can get by with a streamlined procedure, using just a "clean" process rather than a sterile one. No need to swab, no lubricant, no rubber gloves. And this doctor says it's even okay to wash the catheter and reuse it, a big relief since the catheters cost close to a dollar each. I'm now proud (and not at all embarrassed) to say that I can probably self-cath more quickly and more effectively than a urologically unimpaired person can void. Now I can empty my bladder when I choose to, thereby avoiding most potential emergencies (although the occasional surprise rush call still crops up, just to remind me, I guess, that I'll never completely wrench control away from the Beast).

An added bonus is that using a catheter to empty the bladder completely on a regular basis has drastically reduced the frequency of the urinary tract infections that plagued me before I learned to self-cath. (By the way, a UTI can trigger a kind of pseudo-exacerbation of MS symptoms, so this is an essential advancement. Also by the way, anyone doing self-caths should check with a doctor to determine the best procedure to follow regarding cleaning, lubricating, reusing caths, etc. In some cases, it may be imperative to use sterile techniques.)

▲▲▲

PAT — My neurologist told me that the reason we "go potty" so many times in a row is that our bladders don't empty completely. The bladder spasms shut, even if the urethra remains open. So you go to the bathroom, some comes out, the rest remains. A few minutes later, your bladder works again and back to the bathroom you go. This can go on many times in a day or even in an hour.

I self-cath at the times when my bladder decides it doesn't want to cooperate. However, my bladder still spasms shut even with a catheter inserted. Hence, most times I *still* have to return to the potty a few minutes after I cath. But a lot of others do not have the same dilemma regarding the self-cath procedure, and they do quite well with it. Those who find themselves getting UTIs too often may want to discuss this problem further with their doctors.

Even after all these years of witnessing my bladder problems, my family still cannot adjust to my need to use the bathroom a million times a day (well, maybe not a million times, but it sure seems that way).

On my way to the bathroom now. . . .

▲▲▲

CHRIS — I've been having bladder problems, too, and I think I may have to start doing the self-catheterizing thing soon.

Those of you who already do it: How do you know how? I mean, how can you be sure you've put the straw thing into the right place?

▲▲▲

RENEE — Chris, the first rule of thumb on female catheters— since I have no experience with the male ones—is: If you get the catheter into a hole (assuming this is what you meant by "put the straw thing into the right place") but nothing comes out, you're in the wrong slot. If you are in the wrong slot but something feels vaguely familiar, get your male companion to a vitamin store immediately or check into weight-lifting for male body parts the size of a pencil. If nothing comes out but something feels vaguely familiar and you actually like it (i.e., you have a reaction somewhat akin to sitting on the back of a fully revved-up Harley), forget about peeing and just enjoy the moment. And don't worry about whatever Dr. Ruth might have to say about all this—she can't know everything.

Seriously, Chris, I'm sorry you are having bladder problems. I hope you get better soon. And if you ever have to do the self-cath routine, trust me, it's a piece of cake. I wish I had started it years and years ago. I still have a problem every once in a while, if I am half asleep, with putting the damn thing in the wrong hole, which of course necessitates washing it off and trying again. Then, if it keeps happening, I just forget the washing-off business and keep trying till I get it right. So far I have not had problems such as infections or anything.

Self-cath is the way to go, I'm telling you. Of course, I can also still pee the old-fashioned way—it's just harder for me to completely empty my bladder that way.

With all that said (and I truly hope I didn't offend anyone, male or female, with this silliness), I now have to go find my own catheter, which I have fondly named "Flo." Oh, by the way, don't make the mistake I made—don't leave it out, standing upright in a cup next to the toilet, for all the world to see. My neighbor has a five-year-old who stays here a lot. One day, after he went inside alone to use the bathroom (all the grown-ups and the other kids were outside), he brought my catheter outside, waited quite politely until there was a break in the adult conversation, pulled it out from behind his back, and said he couldn't figure out how I got food out from between my teeth, since my "pick" has two little holes in it.

So, be forewarned. Keep the caths out of sight, especially if there are children lurking around.

▲▲▲

KIM — Self-cathing isn't bad once you get used to it. I've done it for about seven years. The worst part is learning your anatomy by means of a plastic tube. Just when you thought you knew where everything was! The one thing I did learn quickly was to use the disabled persons' stalls in public restrooms. The others just don't have enough room for the required maneuvering. I take little homemade cath kits with me everywhere I go. A little Baggie, the cath, sanitary wipes, and a lubricant. If you need to know more, just let me know!

▲▲▲

Kim's homemade cath kit could be modified, items added or deleted, depending on what method of catheterization has been recommended for a particular person. For example, I don't use a lubricant, so I don't need to carry that. I don't use the sanitary wipes on myself, but I have found it helpful to pack a couple of those (or a paper towel dipped in rubbing alcohol) in the Baggie anyway. Many establishments conserve water by allowing only a tiny trickle to emerge from the faucets in their restrooms. That's hardly adequate to clean a catheter. So I rinse the catheter as best I can, wrap it in a sanitary wipe, and store it in the Baggie until I can get to a more suitable water source.

Another "travel hint": Some patients find the long, soft rubber catheters more comfortable than the smaller, hard ones. I'm lucky that I got used to the hard ones right away, and I have found that it's much easier to hide them in even a small purse.

I also made myself a terrycloth "tube" in which to carry a supply of fresh catheters. When I'm at a friend's house, for instance, and want to use the bathroom, I feel comfortable leaving my purse behind and carrying just the tube with me.

But back to Chris's lesson. . . .

▲▲▲

PAT — Chris, your question about finding the correct "hole" when you cath is the same one I asked. It seems there are only two places (in close proximity to each other) in which to insert the catheter. When I first started, I used a mirror for assistance in finding the right spot. Sometimes I did find it hard to hold the mirror—a combination of nerves and lack of coordination—and, since I sat on the toilet to cath and our toilet was located next to a wall, my son (bless his soul) came up with the idea of installing a flexible-arm mirror at "seat height" for me. So, when it was time to cath, I simply sat down, pulled out the mirror, and found the spot. This would even work when I was standing. I'd pull out the mirror, tilt it to the correct position, and proceed from there.

Now that we've moved to a different home, which has ceramic tiles on the wall, I sometimes use books or whatever is handy to prop a mirror on when needed. Once you've been self-cathing for a while, though, you tend to remember the whereabouts of the hole, and by slowly (and gently) fiddling around in the area, the cath will go in all by itself. Of course, I've missed the hole, as Renee has mentioned, and I do use lubricants, as someone else has said. If you need to know more, should the time come, just ask. There are many of us here with assorted ideas and tips on this procedure.

Now that I've written more than any of you really care to know about self-cathing, I find I have a sudden urge to go to the potty.

▲▲▲

DONNA — My primary-care doctor wants me to give the oxybutynin a couple of weeks to do its thing before deciding if I need to start cathing. I've already bought the flexible mirrors for two bathrooms and have most of the supplies I will need.

Gary thought I was getting kinky when I asked him to install mirrors next to the commodes. I hated to burst his bubble, but he was getting all worked up until I told him he'd better back off unless he enjoyed "golden showers," at least until the meds kick in. Bless his heart. His life, for now, is centered around urinating females. Cera (new puppy) and I both dribble if we wait too long. So he has to be prepared to get out of the way if either of us has to go potty. But at least I clean up after myself, and I haven't chewed his tennis shoes yet.

The oxybutynin has already cut my potty time in half, but it is making me so sleepy and foggy, plus my vision has gotten even more blurred. If the sleepiness and the vision don't improve soon, I think I would rather do the cath.

▲▲▲

RENEE — Donna, I've never been on oxybutynin, so I can't help you there. You are so funny. Gary installed the mirrors, and you blew his fun when you explained why you need them? And then warned him to back off unless he liked golden showers? Only you would think of that.

I can't use mirrors when self-cathing. The mirrors actually make it harder for me to figure out what I'm doing. Everything shows up backward, throwing me into big-time confusion.

▲▲▲

VICKI — I had this morning to myself, so I slept late, then got up and ran some errands. Everything was going fine. When Larry came home, I sat outside and drank a beer or two with him (hey, it's hot outside!). All of a sudden I realized I had to pee really bad! So I went in the house to obey the urge. The problem was, I couldn't go. No way. It just wasn't going to happen. So Larry went to get my self-cath kit. I tried to use that, and then realized I couldn't even feel the cath (should I have? I've felt it other times). I wondered if I'd have to go to the emergency room—just to pee?! I finally got the catheter to work. At that point I decided no more beer—the high isn't worth the low. So I took a nap, went back outside, and drank a Coke. Then I came in and peed all over myself. Earlier, I couldn't go if my life depended on it; now I can't stop. It's amazing how many emotions our bodies can put us through in one day.

▲▲▲

KIM — My bladder control has gotten much worse. The medications aren't helping. There's no residual urine after cathing, and no bladder infection. I guess it's just MS. I have started to wear a protective device, like an adult diaper, but it shows through my white uniforms. I was unsure what I could/should wear that would save my dignity and yet allow me to continue to look like a professional nurse. Finally I got some large maternity tops that cover my butt! The boss said that as long as it looked professional, it was okay. So now I have to deal with the fact that numbers of people have asked me if I'm pregnant. I am generally stumped for an answer, but I will come up with one soon! For now I just say "No" and remind myself that at least I don't have to worry about my bladder.

▲▲▲

Deciding to use the adult diapers that Kim talks about may seem like a major step backward (from adult to toddler), but it really is one practical solution to incontinence. When I first realized I needed bladder protection, I was embarrassed to buy them. So I'd buy disposable baby diapers instead and anchor them inside tight-fitting underpants. Then I began to notice that lots of very dignified-looking adults buy bladder-control products (maybe that's one reason they're able to be dignified-looking!). So I joined the crowd, and I haven't been embarrassed since then. These products are more tailored to fit an adult body, and they come in a variety of shapes and sizes and absorbencies. They're much more effective at stopping adult-size leaks than are baby diapers. Depends or Attends or some other such product is a staple in my linen closet now. Sometimes, when I wear one and then realize that I didn't really need it at the time, I think I'm being wasteful. But it's worth the waste, I guess, to have some peace of mind.

Like Kim, I hated the thought that extra bulk would show through my clothes and announce to the world that I can't control my bladder. I've solved that by wearing mostly loose-fitting jumpers, even around the house. I've found a couple of bonuses in that, too. They're more comfortable than jeans, since there's nothing to bind around the waist. And the whole process of rearranging oneself after a cathing expedition is simplified. It's just too awkward and time-consuming to try to stash a used catheter somewhere near the toilet, then pull up underwear and jeans, fumble through the zip-snap-button routine, tuck in whatever's on top, retrieve the catheter, and (finally!) head out. It's much easier to hold the catheter in one hand, pull up the underpants with the other, and let everything else fall into place.

Sometimes we get so preoccupied with bladder control issues that we're even haunted by them in our dreams. I'm glad I'm not the only one!

▲▲▲

VICKI — More and more, I'm finding that "p" problems dominate my life. Lately the problem has been retention. I can feel that my bladder is full, but all I do is dribble when I try to go. Last night I had a dream that the only way I could go was to pee on my pillow... cool, huh? [Poor Vicki! I think this is the third time that she has talked to us about bladder control. Either she's more urologically incapacitated than the rest of us, or she's less shy about talking about it!]

▲▲▲

ME — Vicki, I want to laugh at this (it really is kind of funny, you know), but it's scary and sad, too. I have dreams almost like this. In one, the only way I could pee was to go into church and squat down behind the holy water fonts (I hope there aren't any Freudian implications here, as in "piss on religion!"). Usually I realize, even within the dream, that I'd be able to go if I could find a real john and use my catheter. But I have no idea where either is.

▲▲▲

TARA — I had to laugh here, too, except that the opposite happens in my dreams. I am always peeing, no matter where I am. I can be standing there talking to someone, and there I go, peeing away. I usually think, well, that's okay, I mean, they know I can't help it. Yet I go to extremes to try to cover it up. Or, if I'm not peeing on the floor, I'm spending the night looking for a bathroom. But it's always broken or locked or the stall is too small for me to get into or the whole booth is glass and everyone can see me. Well, that's the gist of it. It's so stupid, yet I dream that kind of thing all the time.

Of course, when I do wake up and head for the bathroom... grrr... there's nothing. It makes me so mad to sit there and think, *well??* If I try to bear down and push, ha! I could pop a vein before I actually go. It's like a game . . . ta da, ta da . . . I'm whistling and trying to relax and to fool the body into actually going. It's like I have to try hard to relax and *not* try to pee before I can actually do it.

And then when I do start to go, it's on, off, on, off. *Then,* when I finally go and think, okay, I'm done, I go to wipe myself and pee all over my hand!! *Okay,* I get through that part, start to stand up, and here we go again. I sit down, nada, stand up, dribble, drip . . . sit down, nada again. Now, someone tell me, where is the sense in all this? (I know there's none to be found, sense in it, that is.)

I do wonder lately if I ever really empty my bladder. That worries me some, which is why I think that maybe I should start doing the catheterization, at least in the mornings. After the day gets going, it's easier. But I'm still never sure when I'm really finished, because if I start to stand up, I go more and. . . . Ahh, this MonSter is really something, huh?

▲▲▲

ME — Okay, Tara, we're back to the cath thing. Yes, maybe you should start doing it in the mornings, and then about every three hours throughout the day. From my point of view, cathing is really the most effective way of dealing with bladder problems in MS.

▲▲▲

Yet we still run into those occasions when it's unlikely that a pill and a pad and a catheter will be sufficient insurance against an accident. Lately there have been a couple of additions to the list of devices to employ when the "rush call" has to be avoided at any cost. One is a tiny patch made of soft, nonporous foam with a kind of adhesive gel on its surface. It's placed over the urethral opening, effectively sealing it off and preventing leaks, at least for a couple of hours at a time. My gynecologist, Dr. G., introduced me to these very recently. I've only used them a couple of times so far, but I've ordered a supply of them, which, I'm sure, will be put to the test often in the future.

Dr. G. said there's also an actual "plug" on the market now, which may prove to be even more helpful than the patches. The ladies in our Froup have joked on many occasions that somebody should invent a "cork" for people with MS and other control-impairing conditions. We had thought we were just indulging in some fantastic wishful thinking, but maybe our wishes are finally starting to come true. Maybe soon we'll be able to engage in previously risky activities (like riding in a car or going to church or wearing a white nurse's uniform) without fear of embarrassment.

In MSers, bowel problems and bladder problems usually act like Siamese twins. I've read that the same nerve system goes to both areas. So, naturally, if one area is getting wrong signals, the other will too. This is all compounded by the fact that the two problems are sometimes intensified by each other. For instance, a person who has problems with bladder control may restrict liquids, which can lead to constipation. Then the congested intestines press against the bladder, causing it to overflow. And then here we go again, restricting fluids to avoid loss of bladder control.

And let us not forget that loss of control or decreased muscle function in the lower part of the body means that the anal sphincter kind of does whatever it wants to, whenever it wants to do it.

▲▲▲

RENEE — Yesterday I had to pick up Dominic's medicines from the doctor, which involves a thirty-minute round trip from my house. Now, I have been down this road a gazillion times; I know with my eyes closed where every store is, meaning I know where every bathroom is. Well, five minutes en route home, I was seized with a stomach disturbance of the worst kind. Thanks to my brain malfunctions, I couldn't for the life of me remember where any of the bathrooms are that the public can use. My muscle tone and sphincter control are shot, so I just drove on in a desperate hurry, praying that I would get home in time. At least I made it to my driveway before everything gave way. Was this funny? Oh, yeah, I giggled hysterically as I washed the driver's seat of my car with Lysol.

I only know of one other thing that's as much fun: trying to prevent this kind of accident by using one of those little enemas before I go out anywhere. Thank you, Mr. Fleet!

▲▲▲

For myself, most of the trouble seems to stem from lack of feeling or, at best, distorted sensations in the entire lower half of my body. For many years I've rarely felt the "urge"; I'd miss the signals sent between my brain and my bowels. I just didn't "know" when I was supposed to go. That would lead to constipation, which sometimes progressed to the point where, with no advance warning, a bowel movement would be horrifyingly imminent. I'm so grateful that, up to this point, my only doomsday events have occurred in the privacy of my own home.

Again, there are medications available for this problem. But my neurologist has explained to me that any drug that helps to prevent bowel incontinence wouldn't go well with some of the other meds I take. I've learned to manage by concentrating on fiber and fluids (lots of fruits and vegetables) in my daily diet, and I follow a routine of sitting on the john for a few minutes after breakfast every morning. In addition, I try not to be obsessive about the whole issue. That, in my experience, has always been counterproductive. And, when it's absolutely necessary, I'll echo Renee's praise of Mr. Fleet. Anything is better than the risk of absolute indignity!

The diaper-type products are again useful here (the full-size ones, not just the little guards), and again if only for the sake of some peace of mind. They're expensive, they pollute the environment, they waste natural resources, they're uncomfortable, and I couldn't live without them!

Some of our folks have taken part in "bowel training" programs, which are helpful in forestalling accidents. The program includes the addition or elimination of certain food items in the diet, exercises to enhance control, and the establishment of regular bowel habits.

Bladder- and bowel-control problems, like any other aspect of living with the MonSter, might slow us down, but we don't let them paralyze us. We adapt and adjust. We swallow the pills that we need. We use the tools that can help. We develop a highly refined personal radar for the nearest restroom, no matter where we are. We laugh and we cry, as the occasion commands. And we try to keep in mind that all human beings go through bathroom stuff at times, whether or not they have MS.

10

And Then There's Sex...!

L. — Are we ever going to get around to talking about some-thing that so far hasn't been brought up here? We're always saying that we can talk about anything at all, because we all love one another unconditionally, and we'll accept one another no matter what, and on and on. And then we never mention sex! A bunch of women get together every single day and the topic doesn't come up? That's unheard of.

I think this issue may truly be one of the hardest with which to deal. The problem is that no one wants to talk about it. Or we want to, but it's embarrassing. Who else can we ask about it, if not one another? I mean, if we ask a neurologist (usually a man), he says, "Ask your ob/gyn doc." So we ask the ob/gyn, who says, "I think your neurologist would know a lot more about the neurological aspects of this problem."

No matter where we look for help, sex among MSers, espe-cially women MSers, is something that is neither widely dis-cussed nor adequately researched. Most of what is done is by men for men. The truth is, if somebody did focus on this issue and found some solid information and possible treatment, I really think it would help to ease some of the physical and emotional difficulties of our lives with the MonSter.

So what do you say, ladies? Shall we do some research and study on our own, and maybe come up with some conclusions that will help all of us?

▲▲▲

L. is right. Sex is a topic that each of us, to some degree, would like to talk about occasionally, maybe even get some feedback on. But until now there have been only rare opportunities to do so. It isn't always helpful to discuss it with friends who don't have MS, as their concerns are quite different from the concerns of those who do have MS. On the other hand, few of us can imagine walking into a support-group meeting of MSers, say, and announcing the most intimate details of our lives to an assembly of strangers who might or might not have the same frustrations or triumphs. We also worry that while their experiences may be similar to ours, they may be dealing with MS on a different level and might not even consider those frustrations or triumphs worth talking about.

As L. mentioned, it's particularly hard for women with MS. When it comes to MS-caused sexual problems, most available literature is directed to males. We see information all the time on therapy groups, injections, implants, and other devices for male MSers who are impotent. We acknowledge that the help is necessary, and we applaud whatever efforts are expended to give a fuller life to our male MS cohorts.

But the time comes when we have to stand up (in a manner of speaking) and say, "Hey, what about us women? What are we supposed to do when we find that we can't function sexually anymore?"

Thanks to L.'s encouragement, we discovered that we have a great source of information and help in our fellow Flutterers, who have been through or are going through it and can share their experiences. In fact, once we opened up, we found ourselves in a singularly fortunate situation. In the Flutterbuds group, we know one another well, care deeply about one another, trust one another absolutely and would never judge one another. We truly empathize with what each of the others is going through in living with the MonSter, including the sexual difficulties it involves. At the same time, the unique semianonymous forum of our friendships has (finally!) allowed us the freedom to present our thoughts and feelings to our comrades and get some feedback, without the need for face-to-face, potentially embarrassing conversations. We can now afford to let go of some of our misgivings and inhibitions. We can relax to the point of having a bit of fun.

For the sake of discretion, participants in this chapter's discussion (myself included) are identified only with a letter of the alphabet (one not necessarily connected to the speaker). Husbands and other lovers, whether male or female, are identified only as Significant Others, S.O.s.

▲▲▲

A. — I've been married for more than twenty years, and I've had MS almost as long. This MonSter has played a major role in my somewhat slow, but different, sex life. I never had a sex life before marriage (I was one of those virgins who no longer exist), so I kind of learned as we went along. My S.O. was the same. As most of you know, it takes a little while before the best of the best falls into place. Just as my best was starting to happen, the MonSter hit. Then I spent many years doing the "pretending" thing. I pretended to have orgasms, pretended to enjoy sex, pretended the whole darn time.

Then the numbness in my body got so bad that I just couldn't feel anything, couldn't enjoy anything, couldn't even pretend anymore. So sex left the picture for a while. I never told my S.O. why; I just made up excuses. He is a dear soul, and he was patient with me. But eventually that patience wore thin, so I tried to do the pretending thing again. Except now a new problem had developed. I had become hypersensitive to touch. This caused me extreme discomfort. I also had increased bladder and bowel problems, and many of us know the feeling of wondering if we will "lose it" during lovemaking.

So there I was. I had nobody to talk to about this because the only other girl I knew with this MonSter had died the year before. I couldn't seem to bring it up with my doctor, and I believed he wouldn't understand anyway. After all, I reasoned, he is just another man, and men have a "thing" about sex. I didn't know what to do or where to turn.

My S.O. started to pull away from me. There was a distance growing between us, and I could see he wondered what the hell was wrong with me. I loved him dearly, and I knew he loved me and I do believe he has always been faithful to me. But in all honesty, I sometimes almost wished he would "get it" someplace else and just leave me alone.

The tension between us grew to an all-time high. I got scared and didn't know what to do. One afternoon, we were watching television and I somehow got the nerve to broach this sex topic. I started out slowly, carefully choosing my words, and tried to explain "just a little" of what I was feeling and why I was shying away from lovemaking. To my surprise, my S.O. actually tried to understand. He was glad I'd said something, and said he'd do whatever it took to help with "our" problem.

We went to bed that night, and I explained where I could or couldn't be touched. Sometimes I'd squirm or push away when he touched me. I was terrified. Yet it was exciting at the same time. Does that make any sense? We spent a long time rediscovering each other that night, in new and different ways. Sometimes I just had to stop him dead and say, "No, don't do that." Sometimes I'd enjoy something. We went through this learning time slowly and carefully. After about forty-five minutes, my S.O. held me close and said if I didn't want to finish the act, that was fine with him. He was happy just to hold me again. I could have cried. In fact, I think I did cry.

I got up the nerve to go ahead, but told him to be prepared to stop at a moment's notice. I told him he could not lean on me; he had to go slowly, as I didn't know how my bladder would react. I don't know how I did it, but we made love that night and I actually had the best orgasm I'd had in years.

Perhaps it was more a psychological than a physical thing, but who cared?

Each time we make love, we have to go through this process all over again. I never know what will be okay and what won't be. Sometimes we have to stop several times just so I can run to the bathroom to "check." I've finally told him all that I'm worried about, and we deal with each thing as it occurs.

I can't handle fast-paced lovemaking, and our foreplay does take some time. It is a very slow process. There are times I've almost fallen asleep during this, to be honest. Not that I am not stimulated, but just because it takes me so long to get that way! No, I don't always have orgasms, but I do have "other feelings" (like super-sensitive areas that have become new erogenous zones!) that this MonSter has given me, that tend to make up for that. Weird, huh?

Well, I'm running out of room here, but I could go on much longer about this. It's easy to talk about once we get started, isn't it?

▲▲▲

B. — I've definitely lived with the sex thing the whole twenty-some years of my "benign/sensory" MS. [By "benign/sensory" MS, B. means that she can function adequately most of the time, but her sense of touch is impaired.] It's also something I've spent way too much time thinking about. But I have come to some definite conclusions for myself.

As far back as twenty-three years ago, I told my S.O. that I felt my body was in worse condition after making love than before. Oh, boy, do I remember his denial as he yelled, "Don't you *ever* say that again!" I remember everything about that moment. He was so adamant! I think it was right then that I lost the complete honesty of marriage, and I realized that the MS was going to change me forever.

Over these many years, I have experienced some things

that I don't mind sharing if it might help some of you who are newer to the MS sex scene. It *is* different—and I am grateful that I had a few years of premarital bliss just so I know what approximates "normal" (although I had MS symptoms in college, too). Please keep in mind that I have a decidedly hyper nervous system, and I describe only my own experience re. *my* body. Also know that I do now and always have loved sexual encounters. I have simply had to alter them over the years as my body responded differently—a very obviously individual thing. I have been blessed with a man who truly loves me, who is loving and giving, and who has chosen to stick with me through all of this. He just still can't acknowledge to himself that that part of our life is affected as much as it is by MS. So it's been tricky, but I have managed to strike a workable balance between truth and fantasy.

Looking back over my many years of living with MS, I can see that I have been through many variations of sexual expression many times. I have seen my share of wonderful sexual highs and lows—more than a normal person, I am sure, because I have had extremes of hypersensitivity (both good and bad) and frustrating times of "deadness" as well. I also realize that I have been fortunate that my ability to reach orgasm is unaffected, when that [ability] usually diminishes in women with MS. But by the same token, I believe that I've managed this because I never once went more than a week or so without an orgasm, and there may well be something to the "if you don't use it, you lose it" adage.

For many years in our marriage, we would spend at least an hour on foreplay every time we made love. After maybe fifteen years, I saw this had to be modified due to my fatigue and extrasensitive skin areas; I began to talk about Plans A and B and C. That meant basically an assessment of how much foreplay I could tolerate effectively, and in some cases, whether we should stop short of "the act." At those times I obviously offered equally tantalizing alternatives. I also helped my S.O. learn when his touch had to be firmer, gentler, etc.

Another milestone came after about eighteen years when we introduced a vibrator into our lives. That was a major breakthrough in that it greatly reduced the amount of foreplay, which translated to less assault on my nervous system. The quicker foreplay with a vibrator, for me, means I can handle really wonderful orgasms without my body rebelling, which has come to be my choice most of the time. In other words, I learned to be patient during my own building phase, getting just enough stimulation to "get wet," and I began to see much of making love as giving more than getting. Because I'm able to "be ready" just by giving, so to speak, I can save all stimulation, if I choose, for another time, depending on my judgment of my stimulation tolerance during that particular encounter.

This arrangement came to be something I preferred, because I knew my "time to come" would come and because I was parceling out my limited resources so that I wouldn't overload. Now that's just what I chose to do; but it speaks to the need to define our own limits and then construct plans that allow for whatever aspects of sex we want and can enjoy, without sacrificing other aspects.

Maybe the best thing is that finally, after all these years, I am able to be honest with myself about the changes MS has made in my love life. I guess that's what acceptance is all about.

This is a subject that certainly needs to be discussed, with honesty and a clear perspective. But then, I think we all agree, it's a subject dear to us!

▲▲▲

M. — I can really identify with your letter, B. I have a few things to share, too. Ten years ago, I had to have surgery to cut a nerve in the lower right quadrant of my pelvic area. It was always difficult for me to achieve orgasm; I never could with intercourse alone. After the surgery, it was even more difficult because I have no feeling on the right side of my pelvic area. When I remarried, my sweet and caring S.O. suggested a vibrator. I was embarrassed to use one, but he talked to me about his feeling bad if I was unable to enjoy lovemaking. I think my kids would die if they knew their mother used a vibrator. But it has really helped us.

▲▲▲

C. — A problem that sometimes gets ignored is the fact that MS causes such confusion about one's "identity," especially when cognitive and emotional symptoms are chronic. Then it's rather difficult to feel at all desirable. Self-esteem is sort of essential for a satisfactory sex life, and I don't mean just an orgasm.

Frankly, I don't really care whether sex results in orgasm for me, but I do care that my husband isn't so preoccupied with the issue that he wears me out with trying and leaves me feeling like a failure, when the problem is just a failure of communication between various components of the central nervous system. When your partner focuses on "performance," the results don't tend to make one look forward to the next intimate encounter.

▲▲▲

K. — I agree with C. about not caring whether sex results in an orgasm (for me, not my S.O.; somehow it bothers me much more if it doesn't work for my partner). I mean, the opportunity is there when I want it; yes, my S.O. and I do use a vibrator sometimes, and it does make up a lot for lost sensory acuity. But even using it is hard for me—it's just another reminder that I'm not the same woman I was when my dear S.O. and I got together. No matter how many times my partner tells me that I'm still attractive and desirable, I always have this little voice inside that says, "Yeah, right."

Also, it's hard for me to get psyched for sex. I mean, all my movements are clumsy and awkward—and even when I'm able to move, I can't trust that my efforts at moving will get me where I want to be. I think, "Who wants to make love with a klutz?"

And then there's the MS fatigue. Maybe if my S.O. could be home in the mornings occasionally, when my energy level is highest, and if those times could coincide with times when nobody else is around. . . . But leave it for night, and we might as well just leave it, period.

Then the medications—necessary to control pain, spasms, and all the other good stuff that this MonSter packs—wipe out your libido and/or any possible sensory perception of pleasure. And of course, that's all on top of the numbness caused by MS.

My S.O. knows that I'm more than willing to cooperate in and enjoy our lovemaking to the very best of my ability. But don't leave it to me to initiate lovemaking. It's just not a big priority for me anymore. Besides, my S.O. and I have found other ways to express what we used to say with sex. It takes some imagination sometimes, but it's do-able.

▲▲▲

D. — What I want to know is, does anyone else find that when they have sex they can't walk or do anything without huge tremors the next few days? When I have sex, I use muscles in every part of my body; they get very tired and I end up with tremors that are really bad, so bad that my legs won't hold me without giving way every other second. My arms get so shaky that I can't even hold a pen. Now my former S.O. was a dear, and tried to help by stuffing pillows here and there and everywhere. The thing is, I get nowhere close to an orgasm unless I tense up the muscles all over my body, and that is enough to kill the next week for me. The muscles are strained and hurt like a bastard for the week, especially in my upper back.

I have been thinking of this stuff lately because it has been two years since I was involved with someone, and I have to consider it should I ever enter into an intimate relationship again. I mean, is being sexually active an option if I also want to be otherwise functional? I feel that if having sex brought me to tears half the time two years ago, what is realistic now? Is it something that I have to forego? How would I make adaptations so that I could still be functional?

Some of you have talked about being numb. I am not, and yet sometimes I think, well, if I was, then I would not tense up so in sex because I wouldn't feel all that good stuff going on and my body would not react like it does and I could maybe control it better. But then, who knows? I am just really puzzled. I think it is important to enter into any relationship honestly, but I don't know the answers here. Of course, as I ramble along, I realize that I am not entering into a relationship now, and this may never be an issue. But I choose to think that it will be.

▲▲▲

E. — I am so glad to know that I am not the only one that has huge tremors after sex. For a long time now (I don't remember when this started), every time my S.O. and I make love I am completely, totally fatigued afterward, sometimes for the rest of the day or even a few days. Plus, my numbness increases every time. I am also one of those who have to tense every part of my body in order to have an orgasm.

Now it takes longer and longer, and then add in the fact that my skin is so sensitive that I can only take so much stroking. Sex has become a process of "Move here" (my S.O. just grabs my legs and slides me around wherever), "Prop up here," "No, that doesn't feel good today. Let's try this." And so on and so on.

I have no problem, nor does my S.O., with using a vibrator. Fortunately my S.O. is not the type to take it personally if I need "outside" help. But I remember reading somewhere about a woman (this has nothing to do with MS) who used a vibrator so much that finally that was the only way she could climax. I think that is what I fear. What if that becomes the only way for me? (Okay, I'll deal with it.) What if it starts taking more or bigger or whatever to achieve climax?

I have learned from all of you that we are all pretty much in the same boat, struggling with the same problems regarding MS and sex. Thanks for letting me know that I am not the only one who has these "side effects" from making love.

▲▲▲

J. — Sex, huh? Okie dokie. . . .

Well, the right side of my body is hyper-spastic (it kind of jerks around on its own) most of the time, and I'm seminumb in all the areas that count. Two counts against me right away! I have found that it takes a lot more stimulation, and I'm talking *direct* stimulation, than it did before MS. I've adapted to the fact that my body will no longer function sexually without aid, just as the rest of my physical body needs aid, if I am to be happy, unfrustrated, not constantly in tears, and sexually fulfilled. I had to be honest with my partner. He's secure enough in his own sexuality that he bought me a vibrator. If that's what it takes, then he's willing to use it. I have a very special guy, and I am very grateful that he is not the kind that thinks he has a "magic wand." We are both aware of the havoc MS can play in any area of our lives. A healthy sex life takes teamwork. So honesty, open-mindedness, and willingness to experiment and to talk openly and share our likes/dislikes in *all* areas of our life together seems to work quite well. (Also, if I'm in the mood and he's not, his joke is, "Well, I bought you a vibrator. . . . It's a cheap substitute.")

▲▲▲

L. — Okay, can anybody help me with this one? My S.O. and I just plain aren't having sex anymore. No, we're not having any other problems. I know we still love each other. We just don't have sex.

▲▲▲

S. — My S.O. and I have gone through that (no sex), L. We are just starting to get out of it. His problem is that he is so afraid of hurting me. I'm going to get kind of graphic here, so sorry if I offend anyone. I have a big problem with lack of vaginal moisture, as in I don't get wet no matter how much foreplay there is! So between his ego taking a blow from that and the fact that I can easily get rubbed raw, he just backed away. We fixed a great deal of that by having lubricant by the night stand, but the psychological aspects are still there. He sees me as very fragile and is afraid to touch me.

It's my job to help him get over that. I have to flat-out tell him what feels good and what doesn't. That's not exactly an easy thing for me, but it has been helping a lot. I'm sure the fact that our S.O.s feel so damned helpless doesn't exactly do much for their ability to "get in the mood" and make things progress further.

My S.O. felt just as stuck as I did, but he was not able to verbalize why he felt that way. Finally, one day he completely broke down and let everything out all at once. It was like a Freudian Vomit! Only thing is, you get one hell of a headache after you do that!

▲▲▲

N. — You hit the nail on the head, about your S.O. being afraid that he's going to hurt you! My S.O. and I have talked about this time and time again. I thought we had worked past this. I just didn't realize how deep this fear can go. Anyway, I do my best to show him I am not fragile. We have to use lubricant, too, have had to for some time.

Although he has made a lot of progress in terms of believing that making love is not going to paralyze me, he always says that he worries about me having an orgasm because of what it does to my central nervous system. It is true—my body is basically the pits afterward, dragging, tired, shaky, you name it. And he mentioned tonight that he has to get past the obsession about what orgasms do to me. I keep trying to convince him that I am fine after orgasms, even when I'm not. That's easier than dealing with his worry. I think that he'll just have to work on that issue himself for the most part.

Anyway, don't worry, you didn't offend me. We MSers ought to talk about this stuff more often.

▲▲▲

P. — N., you were talking about how your body feels afterward, the dragging, tired, shaky, you-name-it syndrome. When that happened to me, my S.O. used to take that as a compliment to his prowess; now it scares him to death. Our problems started way before the diagnosis of multiple sclerosis, when the fatigue was so bad that by the time I did what I had to do, there was no energy for sex. A lot of anger and frustration built up because of that. Then once I got the diagnosis, my S.O. had a lot of guilt for the comments he had made and the general hell he had put me through because he didn't understand what was happening. Well, I didn't understand, either.

We are just starting to get the trust back between us—it was really bad for a couple of years and some life back in the bedroom. He still waits for me to let him know when. I don't like calling all the shots all the time and would love for him to get the twinkle back in his eye when he's feeling frisky. I can remember the days when he would come home from work and I could tell it was going to be a good night.

There used to be a lot of good nights and mornings and afternoons! Those were the days! I'm not ready to give them up!

As you said about your S.O., mine, too, will have to work on this problem himself. All I can do is be open with him about what works for me and what doesn't. I can't accept the changes for him.

▲▲▲

I think we've accomplished the goal that L. set for us at the beginning of this chapter. We broke down the (flimsy, I'll admit) barriers that existed even within the Froup regarding open discussion about sex. My great hope at this moment is that medical personnel and others with the required expertise will also welcome more open exchange on this subject with MS patients.

And then I wonder if the responsibility lies with us to make this happen, too. Maybe it's our own inhibitions that prevent our doctors from teaching us what they've learned.

I'm reminded of something that happened a couple of years ago with my own gynecologist, Dr. G. During my annual visit, he asked how things were going as far as sex was concerned. Now, Dr. G. is one of my favorite people in the world, besides being one of my favorite doctors. It should have been so easy to say, "Well, you know, I could really use some help there." Instead, I said something like, "Oh, it's okay. You know how it is: we have to make adjustments, but we manage."

He patted me on the shoulder, said, "Wait here a minute," and then left the room. When he returned, he handed me a catalog entitled "Sex Aids for the Handicapped." He told me to take it home, use the enclosed order form if I wished, and then send it back.

I did as he told me to, but I only now realize that he helped me with much more than a catalogue that day. Beyond the knowledge that such aids, specific to people with impaired sexual function, are available (and acceptable!), the real gift he gave me was the assurance that he understands. He realizes that sexual problems for somebody in my condition deserve special attention and guidance. He as much as said that he respects my right to not discuss it with him, but that he's willing to offer his attention and guidance if and when I want it.

So why didn't I take him up on that? Looking back, I guess it was because "handicapped sex" was still a taboo subject in my mind. I don't think I fully believed that having sex and even enjoying sex is a "good" thing for people like me. I feel differently about it now, and I'll go to my next appointment with Dr. G. unburdened of a lot of inhibitions. I'll take advantage of whatever counseling he's willing and able to give me.

It has taken the precious sharing with my Flutterbud Sisters, as recorded on these pages, to give me the courage to say that!

11

Sick of Being Sick

KIM — I miss myself so much. I am sick and tired of being sick and tired. I have always been the type to just ignore ailments, but now it's in my face and I can't deny it. When I do, it kicks my ass down and knocks the wind right out of me. I feel like I have no control and am totally helpless. This thing does whatever the hell it wants to me, and I have no say whatsoever. I don't know if I'm depressed, but I almost wish somebody would tell me that I am. At least that way there would be a reason why I feel like the *me* that I am supposed to be is *gone!*

▲▲▲

JAMIE — It sure sounds to me like you're depressed, Kim. Now do you feel better, since you got your wish? I'm kidding, really, and I know that this isn't something to kid about. But maybe it will help you to smile during your depression, if that's what it is. At least you've got lots of company here. We all go through it, sooner or later.

I think depression *is* a common symptom of MS. Our minds get frustrated, and those feelings of "I'm not like I used to be" are hell on us, especially when we have always seen ourselves as strong-willed people who hate to ask for help, would never ask for help, and would never get sick enough to become a "burden" to others.

I am now taking Prozac. I waited until the depression put

me in the hospital before I finally accepted that medications could help. I've been to my own personal hell more times than I care to talk about and *nothing* is worth going back there if I don't have to! And if antidepressants prevent that—then so be it.

▲▲▲

My first experience with a real, ongoing, crippling depression occurred before I had any idea that I had multiple sclerosis. Some months after Karen's birth, I went into what seemed to be an extended postpartum slump, accompanied by other, mostly just bothersome, little signs and symptoms. I had trouble focusing, both mentally and visually; anything I looked at seemed always just a bit "away" from where it should have been, as though I was paging through the coloring book of a child who couldn't quite stay within the lines. I felt exhausted, dizzy, and nauseated much of the time. I had alternating bouts of diarrhea and constipation, and my weight dropped to well below my prepregnancy level. In spite of extensive testing, my internist, Dr. S., couldn't find anything wrong.

I suspected that the strangeness occurring in my body actually originated somewhere in my psyche. Eventually, though he never hinted at it, I assumed that Dr. S., too, had concluded it was all in my head. He referred me to Dr. A., a wise and wonderful psychiatrist, when the depression lingered. After several months of medication and therapy, I felt "straightened out" enough to go through (and enjoy) another pregnancy.

A yearlong span of relative peace followed Julie's birth in June of 1973. I was too caught up with my kids to pay much attention to myself. Some physical quirks remained, but I figured I was still in the healing phase of my earlier emotional problems and that it would take some time to get all the leftover effects resolved. Life seemed very good.

Until the depression hit again, that is, a crushing, paralyzing despair that turned me into a would-be zombie, unable and unwilling to function as a living human being. I dreaded the sight of the

sun rising each morning. I wanted to cover my ears every time
Karen or Julie called. I didn't want to talk to anybody. I couldn't
make myself get up and clean my house, but I felt frustrated and
angry when it got cluttered and dusty. I spent most of my time
(which was all the time that I didn't have to do something for Ron
or the girls) reading, sometimes two or three books in a day.

I couldn't understand my own despondency. My life should
have been the perfect antidote for depression, not the cause of it. I
had a devoted husband, two gorgeous, healthy children, all the
means to keep mind and soul and body together. I kept thinking
about one of my mom's favorite admonitions: "You don't know how
good you've got it, young lady." I almost wished that she would
drill that into my consciousness again, set me straight once and
forever. But I couldn't begin to describe to her how miserable I was.

Shortly after Julie's first birthday, I found myself having crazy
thoughts: "If I walk past that window with one of my babies in my
arms, I'll have to throw her out. I won't be able to stop myself." I
knew that I had to do something. My thoughts and feelings were so
out of control that I was afraid that my actions would follow suit,
and I'd end up hurting one of my girls. I finally made an appointment to see Dr. A. again.

Seeing Dr. A. regularly became a way of life for me for the next
six or seven years. That was a time of "falling into the pit" over and
over again. Every time Dr. A. put me on a new medication or guided
me into a different area of therapy, I'd feel better for a while. Then
I'd plunge again into the depression, with no idea how I got there
and no hope of getting out. I made one serious attempt at suicide,
and the rest of the time I longed to find the nerve to follow through
on it. I was hospitalized numerous times, for anywhere from two to
six weeks at a time. During two of those hospitalizations, I received
electroconvulsive therapy, six or seven treatments each time.

It was in the middle of all this, I think after my second or third
stint in the psych ward, that the "probable MS" diagnosis came

through. During later bouts of depression, people would say to me, "Of course you're depressed; you have this horrible disease." I couldn't begin to explain that I was sure my depression was not caused by the knowledge that I have MS. As far as I could tell, my main emotional response to the diagnosis had been relief. Nothing else changed. The gloom still descended whenever it wanted to, with whatever intensity it chose. I didn't understand it myself, so I couldn't expect anyone else to.

▲▲▲

HELEN — I, too, have a history of clinical depression, mostly from pain wiping out whatever chemical it is in the brain. . . . I just got up, so don't ask me for names. Oh yeah, I think it's serotonin. I've heard that MS hits the same chemical in many people. I can tell when I'm heading into an MS "episode" because instead of getting weepy, I get ornerier than all hell. Prozac helped to "normalize" this and turned me back into a regular curmudgeon instead of a raging bitch. Every time I had back surgery (three, count 'em, three times . . .), I would go through a stage of the weepy, labile, "whine and snot" feelings. The doctor told me that pain of more than three months' duration causes depression, as does anything that messes with the central nervous system.

Grief? Over something like having MS? I don't deal with it. I don't cry unless I'm totally pissed off or if I've just had my back cut open and my spine messed with. I don't seem to run the normal gamut of emotions where plain ol' life is concerned (mainly, I suppose, because I grew up with too much of the "I'll give you something to *really* cry about!" stuff).

It's all part of depression, but it's hard to say what's pain/MS-related, what's genetic, and what's from childhood stuff. I have intermittent bouts of this. It's not always present, or at least not to the degree that makes me need medication.

▲▲▲

Once I learned that I had MS, I had similar questions. I figured that if MS can alter our physical senses, mightn't it also change the way we perceive things emotionally? If it can make a sprinkling of water feel like a dousing with acid, couldn't it also turn a mild, benign melancholy into a ranting, malicious despondency? I didn't mention these thoughts to any doctor back then, though. Even now, many doctors insist that MS, in and of itself, doesn't cause depression. They say that patients get depressed as part of the grieving process after finding out they have a chronic, disabling disease. Or that some of the medications we take can cause depression.

I've come to the conclusion—although there's not much scientific data to back this up—that the real depression (not everyday sadness or regret) we all experience now and then can stem from either situation: the inability to cope with the effects of a chronic illness, or a pure screw-up in the brain's capacity to accurately interpret certain emotional input. Maybe it's a combination of both factors.

It doesn't really matter. It is real depression, not just passing sadness over our losses. The good-news part of this, though, is that something can be done about it. And as with everything else in the MS basket, the symptoms and the treatments are different for every one of us, colored by the accouterments in each of our lives.

▲▲▲

DONNA — I have dealt with the depression monster on and off for years. I have been too stubborn at times to ask for help and have opted to go it on my own. I saw it as a weakness that I just had to get over. I would get angry at anyone (especially my husband and the doctors) who suggested I take medication for it. I didn't want the side effects. I knew I would gain twenty pounds, have a dry mouth, and have weird dreams.

Finally a very special doctor explained the chemistry of depression to me, and I was able to see it in a different light. His explanation erased my perception of depression as a character flaw. Now I gladly take my "serotonin supplement" along with my thyroid and estrogen supplements. I feel better and life is a lot rosier.

▲▲▲

JOY — When I was diagnosed, I was convinced that MS would never be a major factor in my life. After all, I had lived with it for more than twenty years undiagnosed, and I was still going . . . well, if not strong, then strong enough. So I didn't really feel depressed over it. Not consciously, anyway.

Not long afterward, though, I did just happen to meet a therapist with whom I instantly connected. I started crying during our first casual conversation, and followed that with therapy for the next few months. I had a lot of old, unresolved issues, beginning with the accidental death of my teenage brother when I was only three and too young to know how to grieve. So I spent a lot of those evening sessions weeping my heart out. This therapy was extremely helpful, and I was better for it, emotionally, than I had been in my entire life.

I told my primary-care doctor that the therapist had remarked that I suffered from "chronic sadness." This may have been a factor (my doctor makes notes on everything!) in his decision to prescribe Prozac a couple of years later. I told him I didn't *feel* that depressed. But he was seeing stuff I didn't see.

He explained about serotonin uptake, and as he did, I realized that 1) I had been undergoing a difficult menopause; 2) I have a family history of clinical depression, as well as alcoholism; and 3) the MS can affect the ability of our brains to produce and process neurochemicals normally. Triple whammy. And sure enough, after a month or so on the Prozac, I found myself humming as I worked in the kitchen one night, and I thought, hey, I used to do this all the time! I hadn't even realized that the "old Joy" had been missing until she returned! It really surprised me, because then I understood how damned sneaky and gradual depression can be. One of my sisters was an alcoholic and also suffered from depression, and my remaining brother has had problems all his life with both depression and alcoholism. I've been wondering lately how different his life might have been had antidepressant drugs been available when he was a young man.

I'm glad these new antidepressants are available for people like me, who have avoided addiction to booze or crack or whatever, but who still have experienced clinical depression. Which, I'm aware, is *not* the same as having an occasional case of the "blues" or the natural sorrow that comes from the loss of a loved one, etc. I can't begin to guess how many different kinds of depression there are, and I can only hope I don't find out first-hand!

▲▲▲

KIM — I was just sitting here thinking to myself that this disease is so hard to deal with. You have all heard of the Kubler-Ross stages of grieving over loss. I was wondering if we will ever fully accept MS and the losses it deals out to us. Then it dawned on me that with most other diseases or losses, we cope with them, go through those stages, and then we are done with it. With MS, every time something changes, either permanently or temporarily, we have to start that grieving process all over again. That's why this is so hard on us and our families. I'm sure you all already know this, but I tend to be a little slow on the draw!

▲▲▲

I have to agree with Kim on this (that we grieve repeatedly for the same thing, not that she's slow!). The MonSter comes and goes whenever it wants. During periods of remission, it can be tempting, sometimes inevitable, to believe that it has gone away. And it's always a shock to realize again that it hasn't gone anywhere; it's just been taking a break. I've gone three or four years at a time with virtually no symptoms or signs of multiple sclerosis. Then, bang! they're all back at once. It takes some getting used to. Usually, just about the time I'd learn to assimilate the newest difficulty, said difficulty would disappear once more.

I have to say that the first neurologist I saw was less than helpful in avoiding depression-inducing denial. He diagnosed the multiple sclerosis and for years afterward chided me each time I came to him with a new symptom. This was the guy who told me, over and over, "There's nothing wrong with you; you're just too introspective," or "You're just feeling sorry for yourself," or something along those lines.

We can't forget, too, the well-meaning family members and friends who try to cheer us with remarks like, "Oh, doctors don't know everything. I know somebody else who had exactly the same symptoms, and they found out it wasn't MS after all" or "If you'd just go out and enjoy this beautiful weather, I know you'd be fine" or, "There's no way to prove that you really have MS."

And so, somewhere in our minds, we're saying, "Yes, of course, you must be right. I don't have MS; I'm just [hallucinating, shy, lazy, ignorant, ditzy—pick any word or any combination of words]." There is some tiny part of us that tends to believe, especially during remissions, that the relative or friend is correct, that we have nothing more calamitous than a minor character flaw. The next day (or week or month or year or minute), another attack strikes, affecting any number of physical functions. Add in the mixed-up nerve transmissions that cause inappropriate, exaggerated emotional responses, and we end up again with depression.

▲▲▲

SHARON [wearing her Psych Lady hat] — Denial is truly a gift from God, at least for a time; it helps many to survive and to cope with horrific life situations, such as abuse of children and adults, life losses, and the diagnoses of many types of diseases.

I think denial is but one of the many stages we pass through on this continuum. Without denial, people would be unable to survive the pain and sadness which they are experiencing, at least at times. I believe that I have truly accepted my diagnosis. But there are those times that I need to say, "Well, mine is mild, not as bad as so and so's," or "Well, I can still do [whatever goes here]," yadda, yadda, yadda. Let's not give denial a bad rap. It is a necessary function of the psyche and permits us to move forward.

Then there comes the time when the issue we're denying must be faced and acknowledged, which is the only recipe for change in one's life. Of course, there is pressure from outside sources (society, parents, and other loved ones trying to cope with the impact of a child, spouse, parent, or sibling diagnosed with multiple sclerosis or another disease) to deny the existence of the disease. That tends to feed our own denial, to encourage us to ignore the need for adjustments in our lives. I think the hardest thing for me is to push when I can and say "no" when I can't. I think I will always be striving for that ability.

▲▲▲

I went through additional therapy with Dr. A. several years ago to help me clear up, once and for all, denial issues that continued to badger me. Somehow at that point, in spite of needing a cane to walk even short distances, in spite of giving up my job because of the progression of symptoms, I'd managed to half-convince myself again that my problems were all psychosomatic. I trusted Dr. A. to be totally honest with me, to tell me if I really had some psychological disorder instead of MS. No such luck. With the honesty I'd expected, he told me instead that, whether or not I agreed to call it MS, I did have a serious neurological disorder.

Shortly after that, my neurologist (unaware of the things recently going through my mind) ordered an MRI in preparation for prescribing a new drug. It showed extensive areas of plaque in my brain. That should have been the last nudge I needed toward full belief. But sometimes I still wonder. . . .

Now I'm in the secondary-progressive stage of the disease. I don't go into full remissions anymore (I haven't for about seven years), so theoretically I should be alert to daily evidence that this "thing" is with me at all times. Yet when one of the old troubles worsens or a new one shows up, my first reaction is always, "What's wrong with me?" I have to consciously remind myself that I have multiple sclerosis! I wonder if I'll ever be able to get used to that, if I'll ever believe it fully. Will I forever fall back on my "that's not my problem" mentality?

Living with MS is an ongoing, ever-changing process of getting through grief to arrive at acceptance. Every time we acknowledge the MonSter's presence, even during the stage when we're able to view it as a kind of come-and-go phantom, we get a bit closer to finally accepting that *it* is here and plans to stay. Of course, such acceptance means that we may move once again into the depression portion of grief. We have to keep in mind, have to remind one another all the time, that even this is progress! Being depressed means we're no longer stuck in denial. We can't be depressed over something that we don't believe.

Life with MS might mean going through the stages of acceptance many times as the disease comes, goes, comes again, stays, and progresses. The good news is that each time we make it through a bout of denial or depression, we emerge better equipped to deal with whatever garbage the MonSter dumps in our way.

12

Tired of Being Tired

LORI — Lynn, we haven't talked about something that contributes to the depression, something that seems to be my biggest stumbling stone: the *fatigue*. I get so depressed from it, and from my inability to finish anything I've started, much less to start anything new. Then, of course, the fatigue gets worse because it keeps building up, more and more. Feeling so helpless and useless really gets to me. I've always been strong and independent (a.k.a. bullheaded and stubborn), so something pretty catastrophic had to happen to get me down.

I think I am depressed because I am so tired, not because of anything else. I used to be very active, but now I get tired walking from my bedroom to my living room. Many times I've wished for the old me, that one who used to jump out of airplanes and rappel down mountains, the one who feared nothing and was going to live forever and save the whole world in one fell swoop. I feel beaten, not by the MonSter per se, but because I'm not the person I wanted to be. I'm sure none of us "wanted" to be this way, so I know you understand what I mean. I just miss the old me, and that's a bitter pill to swallow.

Sometimes I am so tired it hurts to move. My doctor tries to get me to describe the pain, but I can't; it's not like anything else I've ever felt. Everything is just tired and weak. It hurts when I move—not like a sprain, pulled muscle, or broken bone; it just hurts. I know that makes no sense. If anyone has any suggestions, I would greatly appreciate them. I am hesitant to start any more medications, but if I will become more functional by taking something for the tiredness, then I guess I am willing to try. I think my husband and six-year-old would appreciate it!

▲▲▲

TARA — Lori, I know just what you are talking about, and I too am at a loss to describe it. The tiredness makes everything hurt. Just reaching up to get a box of cereal, I have to hang onto the counter and let the pain go away before I can go on. When I'm really tired, even talking on the phone is painful; actually just *talking* is work. It's like you've been up for three days and your mind and body are just shutting down!

I finally got a prescription for Ritalin. It is a godsend! It's the only thing that gives me enough energy to work. Without it, I would be a veggie on the couch for life! I hope this is helpful to you.

▲▲▲

Some of us in the Froup have S.O.s who, always wanting to be helpful, advise us that it's our computers that cause our fatigue. We've learned to smile and remind them that computers can cause a lot of divorces, too. Then we explain, again, that sometimes we're so tired that our time at the computer is the only thing that motivates us to get out of bed!

▲▲▲

SHARON — It's not the computer! I was tired before I ever knew that the computer on my desk could do anything besides type school papers!

▲▲▲

JOY — MS fatigue is such a bitch to explain to others, or to expect others to grasp. My family and close friends have caught on, but I don't think my boss or coworkers ever did, which is one reason I started working part-time at home. You wouldn't believe the crap I had to put up during that last year or two before I left. People who thought I was the cat's pajamas for years suddenly became resentful, decided I was getting lazy, started finding fault. That was a big blow to the little ego.

It's a subject many of us have struggled with and still struggle with. I think I'll write a screenplay about this, one that people will watch and say, "Oh! Now I'm beginning to understand. Maybe I am being hasty to judge So-and-so. He/she really can't help feeling tired all the time." It's an important topic to me because I was once judgmental (in my mind, anyway) about a friend with MS who was complaining about fatigue at a class reunion, and a few years later, I found that the shoe was on the other foot. Boy, did God/Allah/The Higher Power teach *this* old redhead a lesson! It's also important because we need to get Social Security personnel in various parts of the country to grasp the disabling aspect of MS fatigue and *give us a frigging break!* The rulings at this point seem very inconsistent.

▲▲▲

RENEE — I, too, am so tired, and so tired of it. Everything has to change; we have to make adaptations all the time. What the hell did I ever do to be so fried, everywhere in my body, just because I walked off and on (mostly off) for one hour in an air-conditioned mall? I am trying my damnedest to just function, and that in itself has worn me down. Who would have thought that getting dressed in jeans and a shirt (not even socks!) could be a major production, take forever to do, and then you'd have to rest? There has to be another way to approach this, and I am going to find it. I will not let this MonSter conquer me (even if I'm too tired to remember where I am or why I am there).

▲▲▲

PAT — I had MS a few years before the fatigue set in. It has come and gone ever since. When it drags on too long, I *do* mention it to my doctor, and he checks my blood for a million things. Several times other problems have shown up that needed treating: thyroid, low sodium, anemia, liver levels off, and so on. So if you're ever not sure what to do, it's better to mention it to your doctor.

▲▲▲

I'm always kind of surprised when I "listen" to discussions like this about fatigue in MS. I guess the fact that fatigue *is* a real part of the disease never really hit home with me until I started communicating with the Flutterers and hearing their stories.

All my adult life, I've gone through periods of extreme tiredness, the kind that appears for no obvious reason and hangs around for far too long. It sticks around in spite of extra rest, better nutrition, the ingestion of massive amounts of caffeine, exercise, or a combination of all of the above. As a result, I've seen myself as essentially lazy, unambitious, unimaginative, or maybe too placid.

I spent most of my teenage years in a convent where we were expected to stick to a rigid schedule no matter how tired we got. Our days began at 5:00 A.M. and raced through the hours until 10:00 P.M., through a nonstop agenda of classes, chores, structured recreation, independent study, and prayer. We didn't rest until a bell rang instructing us to do so. We were imbued with the belief that energy begets energy, that there was no excuse for being unable to maintain a productive pace for as many hours as that particular day's regime dictated. Anything less was seen as a sign of the insincerity of our desire to be full members of our religious community.

So, later in life, at the times when fatigue hit the hardest, I blamed it on my innate "tendency" toward complete laziness. I reminded myself that I had been able, at different times, to maintain a very active lifestyle without any ill effects. I knew that it was possible for me to work at my job for eight hours and then come home and cook and clean and do the laundry, chauffeur my daughters to rehearsals, meetings, and social events, lead a Brownie troop, sit at the sewing machine for a couple of hours, and still feel energized. Then I'd do the whole thing over the next day—and love every minute of it. When sheer exhaustion, the kind that persists for days, weeks, months, caught up with me and knocked me on my face, I chastised myself for being such a sloth. I don't think I ever made a conscious connection between MS and fatigue. I just hated myself for being so listless.

Once, when my mom asked Dr. M., "Why is she so tired all the time?" he responded that there was nothing wrong with me except that I had spring fever. This reinforced my idea that I was tired because I chose to be tired. I even asked a sleep therapist why I needed a nap every afternoon in order to make it through the day. She told me that I was addicted to sleep. Another sign of my overall weakness, I thought.

So it's a blessed relief to hear that virtually every person in our group has problems with fatigue. It's even more encouraging that fatigue is now taken seriously as a bona fide ingredient in the MonSter's fare. Studies have shown that the brain requires a larger than normal amount of energy to send and receive information over damaged nerveways. That in itself is good reason for tiredness. Those inefficient pathways also can cause exaggerated perception of fatigue by the person with MS, which doubles fatigue's effects. Fatigue intensifies the symptoms of MS, making coping with them more complicated. That requires using more energy, which creates more fatigue, and the whole process kind of snowballs.

One thing I've discovered in all this is that beating oneself over the head is very tiring. If I forego the self-recrimination and just accept that multiple sclerosis is an energy-zapping condition, I feel much more confident in dealing with the fatigue when it shows up.

It also helps me to pick and choose the things that I want to do. If an activity appeals to me, I think ahead of time about how much stress it will involve and how fatigued I'll likely be afterward. From that point, I can decide which activities are worth the expense of energy and the resultant tiredness. I can also arm myself with appropriate energy-conserving or energy-restoring techniques before, during, and after the activity.

▲▲▲

DONNA — I'm still recovering from a very busy but enjoyable weekend. I spent the whole day in bed yesterday and am thinking about going back to bed now.

Friday, two of my kids brought their families over to swim and play in the pool. I watched the two babies while the parents played with the older ones. After the swim, we reversed roles and I played with the older ones for a while. It was a lot of fun, but I was so relieved when I heard the car doors slamming and the engines starting, signaling the end of the day.

Saturday, Gary and I went to dinner with friends from the police department and their wives. It seemed like old times as we all bailed into the van for the trip. I had carefully planned my treatments and medications so that I could be as mobile as possible yet somewhat coherent. It was the first time in over a year that Gary and I made one of these outings; I hadn't been able to even go out to eat on weekends when I was working. This time, though, I was like a kid at Christmas the whole night. We made it an early night, back home by 11:30 P.M., but I still was exhausted and happy when I collapsed into bed.

Sunday, I decided to go for broke. Gary had to inspect a prospective job site in a town one and a half hours away. The town is close to a state park, some Indian ruins, and several rivers and lakes. It is a beautiful drive and I wanted to go, darn it! So I went! We made a day of it. After Gary finished with business, we went to the ruins and checked them out. Then we drove out to the park to visit a friend of mine who is a ranger there. Then we had dinner and drove home.

This was the best weekend I've had in months and, although I had to spend all of yesterday in bed, I'd do it again. I feel so much better emotionally that it is worth a day or two in bed to be able to enjoy life again.

The old Donna would have laughed at spending a day in bed after such a mild weekend. But I just gagged her to keep her quiet so I can go ahead and enjoy the accomplishment my way.

JOY — I just had to print your letter to show it to Jack. It so perfectly expresses my lifestyle changes and my feelings about them. All we can do is avoid looking back and be grateful for those fine days, even if we have to pay for them later!

It's so good to know that I'm not alone in this struggle!

I'll go along with that!

I used to be embarrassed to admit that I need a nap every day. Now I pretty much insist, at least with my family, that I be undisturbed for an hour or two each afternoon. Sometimes I just sit in front of the television long enough to watch *All My Children* and doze a little bit, or I listen to one of my Neil Diamond CDs. That's all it takes to keep me going for the rest of the day. I stay on a fairly consistent sleep schedule, without apology. If one of my girls comes home for a weekend and invites me to go to a late movie, I usually decline. (However, if one of them ever invites me to a Neil Diamond concert, I'll accept, and then sleep for a straight week to prepare for it!) When I know I have to be up and around later than usual on a given night, I might watch two soap operas instead of one that afternoon.

KARON — Naps are an absolute must for me, too! I've been doing them from 4 to 6 P.M. every day for years now. If I didn't,

I'd fall asleep wherever I happened to be at the moment. I'm so strict about this that I make damned sure I'm nowhere near a dangerous site (like the mall) at that time. And I make sure that whoever I'm with knows not to leave me alone, away from home, after 4 P.M.

▲▲▲

I've never jumped out of airplanes or rappelled down mountains, as Lori has, so I don't miss those kinds of things. I used to stay out all night dancing, work eight hours the next day, and then head for an evening at the mall. I guess I could say that I miss those things, that I'm angry that neurological fatigue keeps me from them. But again, I'm sure I wouldn't try to maintain a schedule like that now even if I didn't have MS. I think that, as Joy says, I'll just be grateful for the days that I can do anything at all, for any length of time, without falling asleep.

I think I'll quit thinking about it and go take a nap.

13

Working Solutions

At the time of my diagnosis, I didn't think much about the effects it might have on my employment qualifications or my abilities to perform in the workplace. As was typical for me, I included "employment concerns" in my list of things that I refused to worry about until it was time to worry about them. Karen and Julie were both toddlers at the time—I hadn't worked outside the home since before Karen was born, and I had no definite plans to return to the work force. I hadn't mapped out what I would do with my life beyond mothering my girls full-time. Ron, too, was happy to have me stay at home rather than deal with the hassles of finding suitable day care for an extended period of time.

But by the time Karen was in kindergarten and Julie was old enough for preschool, I realized that I could go out and "do my own thing" a few days a week and still function as a competent mom. I eased back into a work routine by volunteering as a secretary for a local parish. There was never any hassle about whether to disclose my health condition to management—the pastor, Father C., was a close family friend and was already aware of my MS and what its effects could be. Since I was only a volunteer, I knew I didn't have to worry about losing time or money if I had to take an occasional day off for illness.

Later, Father C. put me on the payroll as a rectory secretary, while my volunteer responsibilities continued in other areas of the parish. I sometimes worked there well beyond forty hours a week; I also got involved with my kids' school activities, became a Brownie Scout leader, went back to college to study writing, and thrived on the whole agenda. When fatigue wore me down occasionally, I closed my office door and took a nap. When other MS symptoms popped up, mild as they were back then, I was mostly able to grab my cane and work around them. Whenever I did have to take time off, it was because of something other than multiple sclerosis.

After eight years, I decided to take an employment break and try to get into freelance writing. I told myself that if I didn't get something published within a year, I'd give up and go back to a "real" job. Before the year was up, I did manage to get my first article published in a national magazine and line up a few other assignments. By the end of that short recess, though, I longed to get back into a situation where I'd be able to interact with other people, face challenges that came from outside myself, and get a regular paycheck to prove that I was doing something constructive.

When I saw a newspaper ad for an editorial assistant for our archdiocesan newspaper, I knew it was my dream job. I had no letters at the end of my name and knew next to nothing about journalism. But, in an uncharacteristically bold move, I typed up a resume and sent it to Jim, the editor. Then I pushed the whole crazy idea out of my mind and took a job in the office of a carpet-cleaning company. My dream, I was sure, had no chance of ever coming true.

Six weeks later, long after I'd made myself forget about it, Jim called and asked me to come in for an interview. Still certain that I had less than a snowball's chance of getting the job, I went downtown to the office. The place felt like home as soon as I walked in. During the interview, I shocked myself by acting as though I had no doubt that I would be hired. Jim helped by acting as though there was no reason why I shouldn't be hired. When I left, I felt almost as confident as I'd tried to appear.

The next morning, Jim called and, as I'd hoped, told me that the job was mine. "There's just one thing I forgot to ask you yesterday," he said while I tried not to shout for joy. "Do you have any health problems?"

My elation vanished. For the first time, I had some idea of what I might be up against with this creature on my back. I saw that there was no part of my life that was safe from this thing, this MonSter. My first impulse was to answer, "Doesn't everybody have health problems now and then?" I didn't know anything about nondiscrimination policies or equal opportunity or workers' rights. I only knew that I had to be honest, and that my honesty would probably cost me my dream.

"I have multiple sclerosis," I said.

Jim hesitated for a second, and then said, "Oh, no."

"But it's in remission, it has been in remission for a long time, and it's never been a problem as far as working is concerned. Even when it gets really bad, it isn't really all that bad, and I just keep right on working." I heard myself babbling and stopped. "Does this throw a wrench into my getting the job?"

Again Jim hesitated. "Not necessarily," he said, "but we'll have to talk about it."

I could tell that he didn't want to hire somebody with a chronic health disorder. At the same time, he didn't want to turn me down because of a health problem that might never show up again.

I grabbed onto this little thread of hope. "You won't be sorry. You know, people with MS work harder all the time, even when, especially when, they're feeling okay, because they know that maybe the next day they won't feel so good and won't be able to work that hard." I was babbling again but couldn't stop. "Besides," I went on, "who's to say that somebody else on the staff won't get sick one day and not be able to work? I'd already be ahead of that person if it happened to me, because I would have been halfway expecting it and would have done enough work ahead of time to make up for it. But it probably won't happen to me anyway, because this disease is so unpredictable, and lots of people just have a few attacks with very mild symptoms, and that's the way it's been for me."

Jim interrupted my barrage of assurances to ask if I'd need to be covered under the paper's health insurance plan (I wouldn't, I said, since I was covered under Ron's) and how I would arrange transportation to and from the office on days when I didn't feel good enough to drive (I'd take the bus, I told him, which would drop me off right across the street from the archdiocesan office building; I didn't tell him that I'd have to walk three blocks from my house to catch the bus).

Jim finally said, "I don't have a problem with this MS thing if you don't. And we don't have to tell anybody else in the office about it right now."

I still don't know if he said that to spare me any discomfort or embarrassment that might be associated with telling the others, or if it was a precaution against criticism of his decision to hire a "handicapped" person. It didn't matter to me. I was proud that, for once, I hadn't backed down and gone slithering off into oblivion as soon as somebody hinted that I was less than worthy of getting something that I wanted. I still had doubts about being the most qualified person for the job. But I knew that nobody could want it more than I did. I vowed that Jim wouldn't be sorry for giving it to me.

I wanted to include here an E-mail from one of our Froup members who had a very disheartening experience when she went after her dream job. (Since she may soon be involved in litigation concerning this situation, I can't quote her words. But I can speak in general terms about it.) This lady, armed with a brand-new master's degree (that she had allegedly been too "disabled" to earn) and enough enthusiasm for ten new employees, applied for exactly the kind of job she'd had in mind ever since she'd returned to the university. She knew she was qualified for it and capable of performing every task in the job description. Her resume won her a phone interview; after that she was invited to come to the office for another interview and to discuss the terms of a possible contract.

When she arrived, she was led to an interview room where she was seated to wait for the supervisor. He came in, talked with her for a long time, and then invited her to accompany him on an introductory tour of the company. As soon as she stood and took a few steps, the supervisor's demeanor changed. His exuberance faded.

She'd managed to hide her hand tremors during the interview, but she couldn't hide her pronounced limp when she walked. That evening, she received a phone call informing her that the job had been given to a "more qualified" applicant. We're hoping that this lady follows through with her plan to bring this to the attention of the courts. We hope the case will be well publicized and will send a message to other employers who might be tempted to base a hiring decision on a person's unsteady walk.

The worst part of this incident is, I think, that this employer will never even know about the assets this lady would have brought to his company. It's his loss, even more than hers.

That sort of prejudice is why I was, and still am, so grateful that Jim decided to take a chance and hire me.

The job turned out to be even better than I'd hoped. My coworkers were a group of dynamic, talented people who shared many tricks of their trade with me right away. I went home exhilarated every day, satisfied that I'd done something productive, that I'd furthered my education more than would have been possible in a classroom, that I'd gotten to know some new friends a bit better. And the wonder of it all was that I was being paid for it.

Multiple sclerosis was rarely on my mind in those days. I felt strong and well physically, mentally, and emotionally.

There was a kind of refreshment in being closely associated with a whole group of people who didn't know about my "condition." I'd been just a bit afraid of how my peers at work would relate to me if it became necessary to tell them about it. Would they worry that I'd use the disease as a way to get special favors? Would my superiors feel that they had to give me special favors, or would they feel that they had to watch me closely for the mistakes I would surely make or the problems I'd surely have? As long as they didn't know about the MS, I thought, I needn't have those fears. I'd be free to go about my business, including the mistakes, as a human being rather than as an MSer.

As it turned out, there was no reason to worry. I "came out" to some of the people on our staff one day after I read an article that one of our reporters had done on a local rehabilitation center that had opened for people with neurological problems. The article stated that the center also had several clients with multiple sclerosis, ". . . even though MS is a muscular disease rather than a neurological one." After some debate with myself, I went to the reporter and said, "You know, your source at the center must have misinformed you. MS is a neurological disease." I went on to explain some cause-and-effect facts about the disease.

She verified the information with the Multiple Sclerosis Society and then asked me, "How do you know so much about it?"

"I have it," I said.

That started a round of questions from everyone who was in that area of the office at the time, along with the inevitable "But you look so good!" comments. I was surprised to find myself discussing the condition in a relaxed, comfortable way, with no embarrassment or fear. Once all the information was out on the table, everyone reacted just as I'd hoped. They acted as though multiple sclerosis was just something incidental I had, like green eyes or knobby knees. It was something to be accepted and lived with on a daily basis. But, as long as the symptoms were quiet, as they were then, it didn't require any further attention.

Another bright aspect of this incident was that shortly afterward one of our managing editors asked me to write an article about multiple sclerosis for a special health edition of the paper. Although I hadn't been hired as a writer, this turned out to be the first of many writing assignments I received in the years to come. This was truly my dream coming true every day.

▲▲▲

JOY — By the time my husband and I approached our fifties, I had invested more than twelve years in the demanding, yet very rewarding, profession of advertising. Over the years, my salary quadrupled, I racked up more than forty awards, and I earned the respect of my peers in the community. I'd worked quickly and efficiently, for long hours, under tight deadlines, and I got along well with other members of the agency teams and with clients. I thought nothing of ignoring vacation days in order to get a job done, and I rarely used any sick days available to me. I enjoyed having disposable income and the little luxuries it could buy, but most of all I basked in the praise and admiration I received from others. Life was tiring, sometimes frustrating, but very good.

When the MS diagnosis came along, I barely broke stride. After a couple of weeks at home to recover from that attack, I gradually returned to regular office hours. The support, encouragement, and warm concern I received from my employers and coworkers made me glow inside. I told everyone what I believed to be true: in my case, the MS would never become disabling, and everything in my life would continue as it had before diagnosis. "Lead as normal a life as possible," my doctor had advised, and that's what I expected to do: ignore the MS, and get on with living.

After all I had read about the relapsing/remitting form of the disease, I expected that any new symptoms—if they arrived at all—would pop up suddenly and dramatically, and after a while would mostly vanish just as mysteriously. I had no reason to expect any new symptoms to be either disabling or permanent.

As I'd expected, nothing happened overnight. There was no abrupt, lingering loss of vision, no limb paralysis, no tremors. Instead, there was a slowly snowballing fatigue that moved like a silent steamroller through my days, chilling my enthusiasm, turning my legs into dead weights, and freezing my thought processes. In its wake came generalized weakness, sleepiness, light-headedness, dizziness, and depression.

When we hired a second person in my position, I began to fight the MS by taking more sick days to stay at home and rest, by shortening my everyday office hours, by virtually eliminating my social life, by hiring a cleaning lady for my housework, and even by hiding in my office at lunchtime and napping on the floor. I began taking Prozac, which lifted the depression but not the fatigue.

Getting out of bed, dressing, and getting to the office (even later than usual) became a major challenge. Remaining alert through long meetings or visiting clients or touring their facilities became almost impossible tasks. After several hours at the computer, my vision blurred, and I staggered as I walked to my car at the end of the day. Even stopping on the way home to pick up a loaf of bread became a major chore.

But I "looked fine."

Some of my younger, healthier coworkers—especially those who continued to put in substantial overtime, and those who hadn't worked with me during my salad days—viewed my decreasing stamina with skepticism. Our boss, it turned out, at first defended me, but she eventually began to listen to their complaints and to echo them. Finally she pointed out to me how many sick days I had used during the previous months. In fairness to others, she said, she would have to begin docking my salary for those extra days.

By that time, I was further worn down by the chilled atmosphere around me and the snide comments I overheard. But instead of resigning, I suggested that I begin working part-time hours at home, and the idea was avidly received.

So my salary and benefits were chopped neatly in half, I used credit cards to purchase home office equipment, and I settled in to work the more flexible hours my body demanded.

For more than a year, this arrangement seemed to satisfy everyone. But it remained a struggle for me to show up at the office as frequently as many people expected. Not everyone adapted well to communicating with me by phone or fax or computer instead of face-to-face. As the agency began to lose business from the clients who particularly liked to work with me, my value to the company, along with my popularity, dropped even more. I once felt like a key player and a favored employee. Now I began to feel like an outcast—tolerated, but not especially welcomed.

The axe fell on a January morning when, during a routine phone call, my boss told me, "You know, we really need to talk about you becoming a freelancer for us or something. I've just hated to bring it up before now." I said that I understood. I had not had much work to do for months; I'd been expecting her to say that.

I hung up the telephone, then sat for a moment and reviewed my options. Over the years, I had known and worked with many freelancers, and I had dabbled in freelance work myself. I knew that it provided a "feast or famine" income and required one to constantly solicit clients and projects. In fact, it involved harder work and longer hours than a regular, salaried job usually requires. There was a time when I might have welcomed the opportunity to be my own boss. But now that time was long past.

The prospect of finding and keeping another salaried job was even more daunting. I don't have the physical stamina for any regular job, not even part-time clerking in some nearby shop.

After so many years of being very employable, I've had to face the hard facts. For the first time in my life, I am not capable of holding down any "real" job. Period.

Period. Such a little dot on paper; such an indisputable symbol of an end.

I'd been at the paper for more than three years when the MS decided it was time to start warning me of my own impending "end." Jim had recently been training me to take over some of the layout and design responsibilities for the paper. We'd just made the final corrections on my first big project and were on deadline to turn it in for printing. I felt both exhausted and excited as I carried the finished pages back to our production manager.

I handed the papers to Rick and, as I turned to go back to my desk, felt a kind of tremor pass from my toes along my whole right side up to my head. By the time I reached my cubicle, my right leg had gone almost numb to above the knee. It was close to quitting time, so I got my things together and headed out to my car. My leg got more numb with each step I took; I had to drive home using mostly my left foot, since I couldn't feel the pedals with my right foot.

I wasn't crazy about the neurologist I was seeing at the time, so I called my primary-care physician when I got home. He ordered a prescription of oral prednisone, a steroid, for me to start taking right away. The next afternoon, he called to ask how I was doing. By then both of my legs had gotten numb and weak, and I had no control of my bladder. He sent me to the hospital for treatment with ACTH, which was given intravenously during the next two weeks.

Meanwhile, Julie called my office and told Jim what was going on. Jim and Kitty, his wife, showed up at the hospital the next day. I held my breath when they walked into the room. I was aware that I'd reneged on my promise to Jim, and I braced myself to be scolded for that. Instead, Jim presented me with a fresh-off-the-press copy of the issue we'd been finishing when the MS showed up. He congratulated me for becoming successfully involved in that area of the work.

"Aren't you mad at me," I asked him, "for breaking my promise that I wouldn't get sick?"

He answered, "You didn't promise that you wouldn't get sick. You promised that I wouldn't be sorry I hired you. And I'm not."

He went on to tell me that he'd talked to the archdiocesan personnel director and gotten information from him about applying for disability benefits if I could no longer work. I was touched and grateful that Jim would go to that trouble without my asking him to do it. At the same time I was appalled. There was no way, I told him, that I'd be applying for disability any time soon. If I had my way, I said, I would be with the paper until somebody had to carry me out of there in a coffin! I had every intention of returning to work as soon as I finished the treatment.

I ended up needing about eight weeks to recover to the point where I could drive myself to the office, work a few hours, and then drive myself back home. In the meantime, as soon as I felt well enough to do some reading and typing, Jim arranged for me to have a computer, along with a modem and an extra phone line, installed in my house. Once or twice a week, Jim or Ron made the trip between the office and our house to pick up or deliver whatever assignments couldn't be handled electronically. Even as I grew stronger and could spend more time in the office, I kept the computer hookup operating for emergencies. It was the perfect arrangement, as far as I was concerned.

I discovered, though, that perfection, or the perception of perfection, isn't necessarily a permanent state. In the months immediately following treatment, my health improved dramatically. Then it hit a plateau and refused to improve any further. I kept waiting for the full remission that had always chased away the MonSter in the past. It never arrived.

I realized then that the MS was no longer something I could expect to deal with only now and then, whenever it took a notion to visit. It had moved in for good. The residual effects of that last exacerbation, the numbness/pain in my arms and legs, the jumpy, blurry vision, the uncontrollable bladder, the screwed-up thought processes, the ever-present fatigue, weren't going to go away.

I managed to stay at the paper for another year. During that time, I had to quit driving; if Ron or one of the girls wasn't available to give me a ride, I was stuck at home. I tried to use the bus, as I'd promised Jim. That worked well on my good days, when I was able to walk to the bus stop in the morning and back home again in the afternoon. After several more months, though, my good days dwindled to almost none. Even if I felt strong enough to get to the bus in the morning, there was no way to conserve enough strength for the return trip. I still used the computer/modem setup at home, but even that was increasingly difficult. I just couldn't keep my thoughts ordered well enough or long enough to start a project and carry it through to the end.

During all this time, every person in the office went out of his or her way to make things easier for me. I knew of times when one of the editors or another reporter covered for me when I couldn't do something or when I did it wrong. I was sure there were lots of other cover-ups that I never knew about. Finally, I had to admit to myself that, no matter what accommodations Jim and the others were willing to make for me, I was no longer competent as anybody's employee. I thought about it a lot, discussed it with Ron, and then went to Jim and said, "This just isn't working any more." He didn't even ask me what wasn't working, so I knew my self-assessment was accurate. We agreed on a date for my last day of work, he gave me instructions on how to apply for disability benefits from the archdiocese, and I was on my way.

I hated to leave that job. Seven years later, I still miss the routine and the people and the deadlines and the challenge and, of course, the paycheck. But deep inside, I know that I did the right thing at the right time. There are days even now that I'd be willing, maybe even able, to get back to doing something, anything more productive than puttering on a word processor. Then I wake up the next day with the MonSter staring me in the face once again, and I laugh at my wishful thinking.

As I look back, and as I listen to other MSers' stories, I realize that my post-MS employment/unemployment experiences have been uncommonly easy. I was able to do work that I loved during the years it was most important to me. I never ran into any kind of on-the-job discrimination related to my multiple sclerosis. When it did come time for me to give up working outside my home, the decision was mutually agreed upon by all concerned. Even my encounters with the powers who confer the right to receive disability benefits were relatively benign. I only had to fill out a questionnaire for the Social Security Administration and another for the insurance company serving archdiocesan employees, have doctors fill out other forms, go through a telephone interview with a representative from Social Security, and then sit and wait the required six months. Both agencies approved my claim right away. This is especially surprising in retrospect because at that time fatigue, one of my major symptoms, was not considered a decisive factor in determining eligibility. (Later legislation mandates that fatigue be considered a significant effect of MS and similar conditions.)

I realize how fortunate I have been. Others have run into harder times.

▲▲▲

JOY — So what does a woman in her fifties, with bills to pay, do when a medical condition forces her to walk away from her life's work? I called our local Social Security office. I was advised to go ahead and file a claim, even though I was still receiving paychecks. So I did.

That was five months ago. My claim was denied. I have filed a "Request for Reconsideration" and am waiting for a decision on it. Meanwhile, my paychecks have continued to arrive from my employer, every two weeks, although I have not been asked to do any work for them and have not even appeared at the office or spoken to my boss since our conversation in January.

That bothers me. I was not raised to accept charity. I dislike receiving money unless I have earned it, no matter how badly I need the income.

▲▲▲

Joy's disability claim was finally approved some months after she wrote about it. The first payment included a sizable check for back payments for the months she spent waiting on the second decision. There's hope even after the big guys say there isn't!

There are times, however, when forced retirement from a loved career involves a loss far deeper than just the financial one.

▲▲▲

DONNA — I was a police officer for six years, and on paper I am still a police officer. I'm just waiting for my medical retirement to be approved. My neurologist told me eight months ago that I had MS, and then said that I should retire immediately because of the weakness and balance/coordination problems.

I didn't listen. I thought I could tough it out and went back to work. I talked with the chief and my captain, who promised to support me in my decision to keep working. At that time I was a negotiator with the SWAT team, a Spanish interpreter, Coffee Corporal (since the guys could not make a decent cup of coffee), and violent-crimes detective primarily working sex crimes, domestic violence, and offenses against children.

Two weeks later, while on duty, I had a major flare-up with optic neuritis, slurred speech, right-side weakness, etc. I have only now started to get some of my strength back. There was no choice but to retire.

The guys have been great to me. They call regularly to keep me posted on all the goings-on. One of them has kept some of my grandkids' pictures that were on my desk and is negotiating with me for their return. He says he will only give them back when I get back to work. I miss that job as much as anything.

They haven't seen the last of me, though. As soon as my retirement is approved, I plan to start lobbying for changes to keep our guys and gals in blue (brown, green, black, or whatever) safer on the streets.

▲▲▲

Shortly after her retirement, Donna's "guys" showed up at her house with a gift check. She wrote to us:

▲▲▲

Just seeing the patrol unit sitting in my driveway gave me a lump in the throat. Hearing the squeak of Cliff's leather gear and the voices on the radio made me want to throw on a uniform and ride around with him for the rest of his shift.

Accepting the check is like accepting that it is over. I get sad and angry that I lost it all in such a short period of time. Eight months ago, I was involved in so many things on the job. I was having a blast in spite of becoming more and more tired and more and more numb. Then, in the space of a few hours, I had to plan my departure from the P.D. and a career that I loved. The reality is that I will never be able to go back to the P.D. as more than a visitor.

I thought I had faced reality, but the truth is that I have avoided it like the plague. I don't want to be a used-to-be anything. I want to be a *still am*, fussing and fighting and cussing when necessary, moving people out of my right-now person's way.

I've written pages and pages about this, trying to understand why I've been so stuck in the loss of my career.

When Gary and I married, he wanted me to stay home as long as possible with the kids. I agreed, and most of my life centered around home and family for several years. I worked part-time jobs, volunteered with the local rape task force, and attended school. When the kids were old enough to be responsible at home alone for a little while after school, I went to work full-time. Then, when my eldest got his driver's license, I applied at the P.D. and planned to fulfill a lifelong dream.

When my youngest was married last year, I believed I had the world by the tail. I had a better-than-average marriage (although I would deny it at times when I was p.o.'d at Gary). I had good kids and wonderful grandbabies. It was finally going to be my time.

Then the fatigue set in and I found myself withdrawing from activities that I enjoyed but could not participate in without paying later. Within a few months, my life consisted of mostly just family and work. I wasn't ecstatic, but I was still pleased to have the best of both worlds. Then suddenly half of that was gone—the part that was just mine. The part of me that I fostered and planned and sweated and studied for. The part of me that filled me with purpose each and every day.

I had reached the spot that I had worked so hard to get to, and it wasn't my training that failed me, or some freak accident. It was my own body that failed me, and there was nothing I could do to prevent the damage or to heal myself of it. There's no surgery to remove the damaged parts; there's no cure. There are just more and more pills to take to cover up a symptom and uncover another side effect. More and more appliances to buy and concessions to make to this damned disease.

On really bad days, I've wished that it had been a terminal illness, terminal but quick. There have been days on which I wished I had been hit by a bus on the way to the neurologist's office on the day of my diagnosis—then no one would ever have had to know about the MS. Then the practical side kicks in and I remember how much paperwork (for the P.D.) is involved in a bus accident, and I know that I wouldn't do that to one of the guys.

There is still a lot of living I plan to do, but sometimes I get so angry that, just when I thought I had the hang of living, I had to start all over with this MeSs. Just when I think I've compensated for the latest attack, a new one starts and it's off to the races again. I know I don't have to explain this to any of you; it just feels good to lose the little Mary Sunshine mask and let it all hang out for a while.

Thanks for listening. I feel *much* better now.

▲▲▲

In the following weeks, Donna got into her application process for disability/retirement benefits. This meant being examined by one of the system's physicians.

▲▲▲

Well, I went for my retirement physical today. From the beginning, I could tell this guy had a problem with my neurologist, Dr. P., and it went downhill from there.

He disputed every diagnosis from every other doctor I have ever seen for any other illness. I finally asked him if he agreed that I had really had three children, or had the doctors misdiagnosed them, too?

He suggested quite pointedly at least five times that I should make a follow-up appointment with him for tests to exclude lupus, Lyme disease, and several other conditions. I told him the tests had already been run and that Dr. P. had the results. He said he could *not* say with any confidence that all of my symptoms are consistent with MS. I asked if that meant he would recommend that I go back to full duty. He said he could not recommend that, but that he would not support the MS diagnosis based on the information he had before him. He said I definitely have a neurological problem but that he thought it's very likely migraine-related. He said that heat intolerance and fatigue are relative issues that cannot be measured, that anyone could say they get weak/tired/confused when they're hot, and that it would mean a hundred different things to a hundred different people.

I finally stopped asking questions and put on my best dumb-guy face and listened to him. My goal today was to get my work benefits, not spend the afternoon listening to an idiot spout his nonsense or to educate said idiot.

I don't know if I will get my disability pay, but I *do know* it will be a cold day in hell before I grace the door of his office again.

I am so angry and confused and pissed. I mean *big-time* pissed. I know what I'd like to do, but I also know that if I stir up anything right now, I can put my small pension aside forever. I know that three doctors whom I respect and trust have told me I have MS. I know that I have experienced symptom after symptom for years. I know that since last fall I have gone steadily downhill, and I know that something is wrong. I also know that I want to whup that snot-nosed, arrogant, spoiled brat, who may have gone to medical school, but who has no idea about being a doctor. *But* I won't. Yet.

Trying to calm down, taking deep breaths, and counting backward from one thousand. . . .

▲▲▲

And she was, of course, cheered on by the members of the Froup:

▲▲▲

LORI — Gee, how many of us have heard this? Is this déjà vu or what? Here I go back on my "Well, no shit, Sherlock" kick. This involves the central nervous system, correct, Mr. Educated Man with the M.D.? And the C.N.S. controls what, Mr. Educated Man? Oh, so you mean it can practically fuck with any and/or every part of my body that for some reason, unknown to you, feels like shit 24/7?? Hmmm . . . wonder why that is? Guess it's nothing, seeing as how you can't seem to confidently attribute my symptoms to MS. Well, Mr. Educated M.D. man, *bite me!*

Okay, okay, I'm done ranting and raving. Donna, I know you don't want to raise a stink, but for crying out loud, no one (and I mean *no one*) deserves to be treated like that.

Do try to remember, though, when your legs feel like rubber, you're having muscle spasms from hell, your vision is blurry, and you can't make sense out of anything and can't get whatever words you are trying to say out of your mouth, that you are simply having a migraine. Oh, Donna, darlin', I'm pissed right along with you and I am on the warpath. You ought to tell this butthead he's going to suffer the wrath of the Flutterbuds. And I'm going to be first in line!

▲▲▲

I think that the decision/application process is, thankfully, at least a bit easier for many of us. More along the lines of Chris's story:

▲▲▲

Something really neat happened today! You all know that I left work in March. Well, I used to order all my Avon from a really nice lady there. Today in the mail I received the last order that I had put in, which I thought I'd never get. She sent it to me saying she missed me a lot and that it was a get-well present. I used to work with a group of really nice ladies, and it feels so good to know that they are still thinking of me. God, if I didn't have this @%$#& MonSter, I would go back there in a minute. I guess that's never going to happen! At the end of this month, I'll go on long-term disability, so I'll probably have to go in and fill out the paperwork. I will see everyone there for probably one last time, and that's going to be hard.

▲▲▲

And later:

▲▲▲

Well, I called Social Security this morning to start the process. I couldn't believe the information that they needed! They even wanted to know about my ex-husband, and I sure as heck don't want to get him involved. I said that I haven't seen him in about eighteen years. Anyway, I am going to get a call at 8:15 in the morning (yuck) on September 9, and then I can mail in all the information. I called to get a copy of my birth certificate, and they can't find one! I guess I don't exist! Social Security even wants to see my vehicle registrations, my life insurance policies, tax assessments on my house, and the list goes on and on. I was ready to tell her how many times a day I go to the bathroom! I don't know if I can do this, guys. I'm really going to need your help!

▲▲▲

DEE — You really have to play their [Social Security representatives' and insurance claims people's] game. Explain your limitations as completely as you can. If they think you are able to walk to a bus stop, they will probably deny your claim. So when they ask how far you can walk, answer something like, "Some days I can walk to my mailbox and back; other days I have trouble making it to the bathroom." There are no innocent questions. They all have some underlying motive. When they ask you anything about your limitations, try to imagine why they want the information (how they might use it to deny you). Then be honest, but tailor your answer to that possibility.

▲▲▲

A few days later:

▲▲▲

CHRIS — I had my SS call this morning and it went pretty well. Just one mistake: When she asked me what my disability was, I went into the symptoms and didn't even remember to say I had MS! I'm sure she'll see it on the reports I sent in. She said I probably won't hear anything for about four months. They sure take their time, but she did say that I did a good job! I was lucky to get three hours of sleep last night, because I was worrying so much. It looks like it turned out okay! I'm glad it's over!!

▲▲▲

A few months after Chris wrote this, we found out that it really did turn out okay. Her claim was approved, requiring no further documentation, no additional doctors' exams, no court hearings. Way to go, Chris!

There are, of course, some who are able (or enabled) to continue to hold down a job well into their lives with the MonSter.

▲▲▲

TARA — I've had MS symptoms for more than twenty years. Other than some minor weakness in my arms and neck (and oh yeah, that fatigue!), I really didn't have too much trouble through the years that I couldn't handle while continuing to work. In the past two years, my MS has turned progressive. I've slowed down a bit physically, but I still go full speed ahead in my job.

Our local vocational rehabilitation center has helped so much. They bought me an electric chair and are putting a ramp on my house, they have plans for renovations to make my kitchen and bathroom wheelchair accessible, and we are working on getting the van that I need. They will turn somersaults to keep you out there working.

▲▲▲

The school where Tara works cooperated in efforts to keep her on the job by making changes in her schedule and allowing her to do some of her work at home. Also, after some negotiation (and some education about the heat sensitivity of MSers), school officials installed an air conditioner in her office.

▲▲▲

TARA — The whole school is getting an education in MS. Most of the people there think it is just something that para-lyzes you, and that's it. But they're seeing that I have good days and bad ones. One of the teachers saw me moving at a pretty good speed down the hall yesterday and said, "You're moving fast today. Good day?" I was so proud of her! These people have gone through the breathing problems with me, they have held me up through the terror of some symptoms that I was sure would kill me, and they have laughed with me at the tremors that cause me to spill everything that I touch. I'm very happy to see so many people come to such a good understand-ing of this disease. They still expect the highest-quality work from me. Yet they roll with me and tend to things if I need to be at home recovering from a hard hit. It has been great!

You have to choose your battles. I choose to work because that's what I enjoy doing. Others may choose to stay home and tend to the housekeeping and kids and that end of things. It really depends on what you are happy doing and what you are capable of doing. Don't give up your dreams because others tell you that you can't do something. Go for what is good for you, and if you need help, ask for it.

14

Earrings and Old Man's Cave

One morning recently, I was getting myself together for the day. I dressed, put on my makeup, and fixed my hair. I'd recently cut my hair short, and I decided I needed some kind of accessory, earrings maybe, although I rarely wore them just around the house. So I got a pair out of my jewelry box, sat down in front of the mirror, and tried to put them on.

My vision was blurred, so I had a hard time seeing the holes in my earlobes. I took my glasses off and tried again. That didn't help. I poked around blindly for a few minutes, then tried to locate the hole by touch. As usual, my fingertips were too numb to feel much of anything. So I teamed up my distorted sense of sight and my muffled sense of touch to search again. I finally found it, kept one finger on it, picked up the earring, and went for it. My aim was way off; every time I tried to slip the post into the opening, it hit just off center. By the time I got it where it was supposed to go, my earlobe was sore, even bleeding a little bit. But it was in there! I held it in place and tried to pick up the little thingy that goes on the back to keep it on. My fingers wouldn't grasp—they just kept shoving the back piece around on the table. I did get ahold of it a couple of times, but I couldn't turn it over to get it into position to slip onto the post, and I dropped it again while trying. After about ten minutes, my arms were tired from holding my hands up to my ears, my earlobe had a sticky scab forming around the earring hole, I still couldn't get the earring hooked up, and I was in tears.

I looked back into the mirror. You're pitiful! I thought. You have, at one time or another, lost the ability to walk, to see out of both eyes at the same time, to swallow without choking, and to move your left arm. And you're crying about not being able to get a damned earring in place? Get a grip!

But I couldn't talk myself out of it—I still felt like crying, because I still couldn't get the earring in. I usually don't cry easily, so I wondered what was going on, why I was so affected by such a small "disability." It occurred to me then that when I do end up in tears, it's almost always because of something that, all by itself, should have meant next to nothing.

I guess I have major problems dealing with the small, individual components of the bigger adjustments I've had to make. Like catheterizing—once I learned how to use a catheter and started doing it (on doctor's orders) on a regular basis, I had no problem with the whole big idea of needing help to do something as basic as emptying my bladder. But I absolutely hate to do it in a public restroom, where the sinks are in a separate area from the commodes. That always means that, after the bladder-emptying routine is performed, I have to juggle the cath (don't want to put it back in my purse or lay it down just yet, can't hold it between my teeth) while I put my clothes back together. Then I have to carry the cath out to the sink area, where there might be half a dozen people to watch me wash it off before I return it to my purse. If I think about it realistically, I realize that there's little chance that anyone will even notice what I'm doing. If they do notice and ask what it's for, I'll tell them. If they look at me funny but don't ask, then let them be curious. No matter what happens, it's no harm to me or to anyone else. It's such a small concern. But I hate it.

I remembered an incident several years before, at a time when walking more than a hundred feet started to be difficult for me on an everyday basis. A friend of ours from Italy was visiting, and Ron and I decided to take him to explore a group of caverns in a state park a few hours from our home. We'd been there before, many times, and loved it, so we were eager to share the beauty of the place with our friend. We made all the arrangements for a good departure time and the supplies to pack for the hike through the caverns, and found someone to feed our dogs late in the day. Then I realized . . . there's no way in hell I can walk through those caves anymore. And wheelchair accessible? Not likely, considering that when we were there before, we spent a lot of time climbing over rocks, jumping over streams, and squeezing through tunnels just to stay on the trail. I'd never really gotten upset over the general fact that my walking ability had deteriorated, but it devastated me to realize that I couldn't hike through Old Man's Cave anymore!

I remembered that on the last several occasions when I reached for a particular bottle of spices in the rack or a specific bottle of pills in the cabinet, I knocked off two or three of the other items on the shelf. I could see exactly where I had to aim with my hand, but I couldn't get my brain and my hand to track with each other. I pictured myself having to "store" all my bottled medicines and cooking supplies on the floor, since that's where they all ended up every time I wanted one of them. The image should have been at least slightly humorous, but I found it depressing, again to the point of tears.

I remembered the last two times I sewed a jumper (my usual uniform) for myself. I breezed right through the construction of the clothing, but I couldn't figure out how to sew on the buttons and trims. I felt so frustrated that I was ready to throw away the almost-completed piece on which I'd worked so hard, just so I wouldn't have to deal with holding a needle and maneuvering it through the buttons and fabric.

I wondered if I was petty and narrow-minded to be so distressed about things that should have had no significance: earrings and Old Man's Cave, and spices and buttons and bows, and all the other small stuff. So I asked the ladies in our group how they felt.

▲▲▲

BARB — That's it, Lynn. The earring thing is a *big* thing. Our dexterity seems to have moved to Des Moines—and left us behind. I have not had long, hard exacerbations, and I feel petty for complaining. But overall, the little things have added up to be one big pile of *I'm mad as hell and I can't take it any more!*

▲▲▲

VICKI — I quit wearing earrings for the same reason. I can't put them on without help from my daughter. I can ride my scooter/wheelchair without a thought when I have to, but I get pissed when I can't tie my shoes.

I very seldom buy shirts that don't pull on. If I do get one that has buttons, I *never* unbutton them. I slip them over my head, too. I wear very little jewelry. Too hard to clasp.

Who was it that said, "Don't sweat the small stuff?" They never had the MonSter visit them. None of it's small stuff!

▲▲▲

DONNA — I think I know what you mean about the little things that are so aggravating. I have always had long, well-manicured nails, which I have kept shaped and polished to perfection. For years, I could almost do them blindfolded. Never had to worry about smudges or smears. I could polish my nails in the car on the way to church and never get a drop out of place. Now I have to have every light in the room on and prop both arms on something, and the hand being polished has to be flat on the table or counter. Between the shakes and blurred vision, it has become a very difficult and frustrating task to complete.

I miss the walks in the woods and exploring, too. My grandparents own the farm where I was raised, and they, my parents, and my brother still live there. There are hills and creeks and ponds all around, where I wandered and roamed and climbed and waded as a child. I took my kids through the rounds several times each year as they were growing up. The last time I went home for a visit, I had the urge to go exploring again, but I knew I couldn't climb over the first fence to just get into the pasture, let alone walk the fields. I can get around on the four-wheeler, but it isn't the same as walking through the leaves and pine needles. The smell of gasoline contaminates the smell of nature.

Since the peeing problem—too little, too often—has hit in full force, I've had to start choosing my clothes according to ease of removal. I don't wear shirts that tuck in, or belts, since by the time I get everything in place it's time to go again. I have seriously considered putting snaps in the crotch of my pants just to be able to pop and go. But then again, I've wondered how much coordination would be required to resnap them and line the snaps up properly before leaving the bathroom. So I guess I'll just keep wearing dresses when I leave the house. Which means I have to shave my legs more often, which is another problem entirely.

Yes, Lynn, the little things are definitely irksome. But there are so many other little things that make life worth living and that make us who we are. I think it's because we consider the little things no-brainers that we are offended when we lose the ability to perform them, because the changes chip away gradually at who we are. When we get around to taking inventory of the changes we have gone through, we realize that the no-brainers require more effort than they should and we get pissed and/or sad and/or scared and/or take it inside and let it eat at our self-esteem.

▲▲▲

LORI — *Yup!* Boy, did you totally hit it on the head. It is the little things. I'm great at handling the crises, but the little things, forget it! I, like you, am hard to drive to tears. When those little things happen, I usually draw inside myself and hide so that no one can hurt me. Makes no logical sense, I know, but then MS isn't logical, now is it? The little things send me into the deeper depressions. When I visited my parents in Florida and we went to the parks and did the tourist thing, they got an electric cart for me. Now, being twenty-eight and having, I'm sure, all the vanities a twenty-eight-year-old still must have, I thought this would truly bother me. Well, it didn't—not one little bit! I had an absolute ball and actually got to enjoy what we did instead of dragging myself all over hell's half-acre and feeling miserable.

Then Steve and I went to see *Air Force One* on opening day (whenever that was). It is an incredibly tense movie; you are on the edge of your seat the entire time. When it was over and we got up to leave, my legs would not stop shaking. I couldn't go anywhere. I knew it was just because I had been so tense during the show. A small thing, but oh, how that bothered me!

Those who are new to this disease should be forewarned that it's the little things that will sneak up and get them when they least expect it. Maybe they should prepare themselves ahead of time, so that when a little thing hits them in the head, they can say, "Okay, they told me this was going to happen. I'm going to be all right."

Donna, you said that you're thinking about putting snaps in the crotch of your pants. Now that just might be something I'd pay admission to see! There's not a chance I could resnap them without having to turn myself completely upside-down, totally ruining whatever mess it was I managed to arrange my hair into and smearing lipstick all over my clothes. No siree, no snaps for this one!!

As for shaving your legs, aw, the hell with it! Let's move the Fogbound Ranch to Europe and just forego all shaving. Or we could outlaw shaving on the ranch altogether, no matter where it ends up being!

Yeah, I had a little thing happen today. My sister took me out to one of the local buffets. I was feeling so good because I had finally gotten some sleep. I totally forgot about everything else. Just for one little split second, I actually felt normal. Then, as I was going through the dessert bar (of course the most crowded), I grabbed the tongs to get a brownie and lost control of my right hand. It really was funnier than hell. Brownies were flying everywhere! Some might consider that pure paradise. But it was one more little thing that reminded me there's something wrong. These strange little uncontrollable things happen when everyone is looking and there is no "logical" explanation for the incident as far as others are concerned, other than that you're drunk, stoned, or just clumsy and stupid. After all, "you look just fine!"

▲▲▲

BREN: What I miss *horribly* is being able to pick up my children. Now, they *are* eight and eleven. But I remember hefting my nieces and nephews at those ages and tossing them around. I can't even pick my own kids up when they're hurt. That kills me.

Okay, that's enough. It may not seem like a big thing, but it hurts to say it or even think it. So now I will put that "can't" back where it was, and concentrate on the "cans." And thank the good Lord that I can still hug my children, see them, talk to them, have an influence in their lives, swing on swings with them, take them to the YMCA, watch them swim, kiss those boo-boos, and put on numerous Band-Aids. Not to mention tuck them in at night and kiss them soundly!

▲▲▲

KIM: I hate when I stagger into whomever I'm with or, even worse, into other people in the grocery store checkout line!

I hate trying to present an idea to someone at work or at home and being unable to find the words.

Or having to go to the bathroom, one of the few times you think you have some control. And someone has decided to move in ahead of you and you pee in your pants . . . or worse yet. . . .

🔺🔺🔺

PAT: Lynn, you mention little things that get you down. I find them to be more little things that I *hate*. Perhaps "hate" is too strong a word, but I do hate it when:

— I'm talking on the phone and can't stand the feeling of the receiver next to my ear;

— My skin is itching like crazy and I scratch and even bleed at times, yet I can't feel the scratching, and the itching won't stop;

— I have to wash my hair at the kitchen sink because if I close my eyes in the shower, even when sitting down, I get dizzy;

— I'm in the mood for sex, but the sensations my skin sometimes has when I'm touched drive me so crazy I have to "pass";

— I'm unable to wear shoes with heels because I'd really lose my balance!

— I'm trying to blow-dry my hair, but one hand can't hold the brush in the right spot while the other hand aims the dryer. In other words, my hands just don't get along with each other;

— I look out the window at the car parked in the driveway, thinking what a nice day it is for a trip to the store. Then I remember I can't drive anymore;

— I'm sitting on the beach and watching the waves rush into shore, longing to run into the ocean, yet I know that one knock of a wave and I'll be yelling for the life-guard;

— I feel the numbness in my legs get worse as I'm walk-ing through a store, and I wish I could just smack myself a few times and get the feeling back;

— I have to call for help when I'm cooking and I can't lift the pot;

— I'm unable to visit my niece's apartment because it's on the third floor and I can't make that climb;

— I always have to use an elevator because I can't keep my balance on an escalator;

— I clip my toenails after a shower and get severe pain in one of my toes the next day because I cut the nail too short but didn't feel it;

— I can't dance a "fast" dance;

— I get a painful steroid shot that should just hurt for a second, but because I get "delayed reactions," the pain shows up out of nowhere a couple of days later and lasts forever.

I also hate that I can't ice-skate anymore; I'm unable to hold a new baby for fear I'll drop her (for real!); and every time I buy a purse, I have to make sure it has lots of compartments because I need room for all my meds and cath paraphernalia.

I could go on with this for a while longer, but I guess you get the picture. Put me in a wheelchair and I adjust, though grudgingly. Give me vision problems and I get upset, but some-how I go on. It seems I can "fight the big fights," but if I drop a glass because I couldn't feel it in my hand, I'll cry my eyes out.

And that reminds me of one more thing that gets to me . . . dropping a glass in the sink and having no conception of what I've done or how to remedy the situation. All I can do is yell for help. Paper cups have their place, but it's not the same when you "have" to use them.

Guess I'd better end this before I start to cry. So, hey, God, while you're helping me with the big stuff, could you maybe lend a hand with these "little" things? Or send an angel or two to help me out? I'm not fussy. Any help will do. Oh, and thank you for my Sisters here. Are they, just maybe, the angels I am asking for, and instead of a couple, you've sent me a bunch?

▲▲▲

RENEE: Pat, re. the Little Things. Your message broke my heart. I know just exactly how you feel.

I sit up here in the loft and type, and after a while I cannot stand it if my pinky finger touches the mouse pad when I move the mouse. Yet I have no feeling in the pads of my fingers. So how can something feel horrible if you can't feel stuff? I don't understand this.

Purses with compartments—I have driven myself absolutely crazy over finding a purse with the right compartments. You would not believe the number of stores I have dragged Marla (best friend) to in the quest for the correct purse. It must have a zipped top, outside pocket, small pocket inside that zips. It must *feel okay* when I touch both the inside and outside material. It absolutely cannot have two zippered compartments that open from the top. That immediately scrambles my brain, and I literally cannot function with the purse.

Materials—this changes every day. Certain materials make me cringe like fingernails on a chalkboard, yet that same material may be okay tomorrow.

Wearing heels—gone forever. The first time I put mine on and realized it was not a good idea, I went to pieces. I felt like I had been slapped in the face. There was this voice saying, "You can't do this anymore." Same with earrings. Marla is constantly having to do my earrings. And sometimes just plain dress me, especially if there are buttons.

Itchy, tickly skin—I scratch till it bleeds. Even spend all day trying over and over to get the "invisible thread" that is somewhere inside my shirt. I know it's there 'cause I can feel it tickling—but it isn't there. Put on a different shirt—presto! there's the thread again.

Smacking legs—I hate feeling that I have to smack my legs to get the numbness to knock it off! I have actually done that; do you have any idea how people look at you if you stop in the aisle, bend over and look down, and smack your legs and tell them to "come on, knock it off"?

Losing stuff constantly—I can't even begin to explain how bad my memory is (forget short-term; we have surpassed that into *What did I say less than five seconds ago?*).

Saying the wrong word all the time, or not being able to form the word with my mouth (brain tells mouth word, mouth ignores brain).

Can't put on makeup—Why? Because the undersides of my fingers have no feeling.

Can't flip through a stack of papers. Can't type some days. Can't feel anything I touch.

▲▲▲

HELEN: Yes, yes, and yes. It's those damn little things that'll get you every time. I remember the worst one for me. My dachshund, Maggie, was a pup about five or so months old. I was sitting with her and petting her, and I started bawling because I couldn't feel her fur! She's almost nine now, so this must have been well over eight years back, but I can still remember the godawful pain I felt when I realized that I couldn't even enjoy the texture of her hair.

And, jock itch. Friggin' jock itch. I have to wear incontinence pads all the time; they don't really "breathe," so I constantly have it. I just hope nobody at the drugstore thinks I'm harboring a gigolo when I go to buy the powder.

Not being able to hold a needle to sew on a button.

Getting dizzy on escalators.

And it goes on and on and on. It's not always the big issues, because they come up and slap you right in the face. It's these little niggling things that, one at a time, aren't bad, but when added together over a period of time seem to just erode my well-being, physical *and* mental, and make me feel like "a cripple.". . .

Or, as Buddy [Helen's newest canine friend] would say, "It's da shitz!"

▲▲▲

SHARON: How about when some perfect stranger asks why you're limping? I always say it's an old athletic injury. There are days when it really hurts to hear that kind of question and days when I am empathetic to the person who questioned or commented. The days when I answer "I have multiple sclerosis" are usually the ones when I have an underlying sadness or anger about the disease going on in me. My frustration tolerance level has dropped to about a minus-five lately. Limping just doesn't get the job done anymore, especially if I'm in a hurry. That probably makes me limp more, which makes it even more obvious that something's wrong. Is this really a "small thing"?

▲▲▲

There are still other "small things that bug big," picked up from random E-mails:

— Wanting to scramble into an interesting-looking ravine at a state park, but not being able to navigate the uneven ground to look over the edge;

— Going down the stairs holding onto the walls and turned sideways, when I could take them two or three at a time a few years ago;

— Having to get up at 6:30 A.M. to be at work at 9:30 A.M. because it takes that long to get "put together";

— Not being able to ride a horse anymore;

— Not being able to drive a car anymore;

— Not being able to balance on a bicycle;

— Not being able to open jars—worse, not being able to reach up to get a jar. Not being able to cook by myself because I can't move the pots and pans around;

— Having to spend most of the summer inside because the heat outside is so debilitating, and then having to spend most of the winter inside because the ice on the sidewalks might be even more debilitating.

A couple members of our Flutterbuds Sisterhood were hesitant to include our admissions about the "small stuff" in these musings, for fear that we'd come across as a bunch of petty, pessimistic whiners. But when I posted my question to the group, I got a tremendous response, with virtually all of the respondents saying, "It's so good to be able to finally talk about this stuff." It seems that intolerance for the little things that plague us is a bona fide big thing for people with MS. I can imagine it's that way, too, for non-MSers who, for whatever reasons, find themselves losing the ability to function at a "perfect" level all the time. It's just easier to cope, at least in the long run, when we're dealing with more monumental changes.

I guess that's at least partly because when big things hit, like being unable to walk or see, our complaints are "sanctioned" by ourselves, by family, by medical personnel, and by society in general.

People rush to help us get through the *big* bad times. Plenty of resources and services are available to deal with ongoing, life-changing things. But when some little something pops up, what are we supposed to do? Call the doctor and say, "Please send me a prescription right away! My fingers are too numb to pick up my earrings!"? Or call the Multiple Sclerosis Society and ask, "Can you arrange for me to see an occupational therapist so I can learn to aim for and grab just the one bottle of spice?"

I'm not at all concerned that anyone will see us as whiners. I think we have a right, even an obligation, to let other people in on the reality of day-to-day life with something like multiple sclerosis. It takes a lot of tiny brushstrokes to paint a big picture. And life with MS is one of the biggest pictures I've ever tried to paint.

I think all of us, with or without MS, learn along the way that dealing with (including grieving over) the small losses ultimately helps us to accept the bigger changes and challenges that confront us, and to still survive as human beings.

15

The Spiritual Side

When a person is diagnosed with a catastrophic illness, it's natural for her to ask God (or her personal Higher Power, whatever/whoever that is), "Why me? Why was I chosen to have this disease?"

I didn't have to wonder. During one of my first exacerbations, my spiritual director at the time, Father P., came to the hospital to visit me. Mary, a classmate from my convent days, was already there when he arrived. Mary and I had been discussing the fact that several of our "former nun" friends had encountered some critical life challenge shortly after leaving the convent. One had gone blind; one had married and was deserted by her husband on her wedding night; Mary herself had given birth to a mentally handicapped child. And there I was, with a diagnosis of multiple sclerosis.

Father P. listened quietly as we finished our conversation. As soon as Mary left, though, he spoke. "You seem surprised about what happened to your friends and what is happening to you now. Isn't it obvious what's going on? You've each ignored your call to serve God as a member of a vowed community. You turned your back on him when you decided that you didn't have to be a nun. This sickness, like your friends' bad fortune, is a reminder that God is still in charge. I'm sorry that you have multiple sclerosis, but it's your own fault for assuming that you knew more than God about what's best for you."

I tried to ignore the words; I concentrated instead on ripping the petals, one by one, off a bouquet of carnations that Mary had brought, watching them drift from my fingers into the wastebasket beside my bed. Father P., though, had to be sure that I'd gotten the real meaning of his "revelation."

"Didn't you also decide, not long ago," he continued, "that you didn't even have to stay alive if you didn't want to? That you could make that decision instead of leaving it up to God? You were ready to let a bottle of tranquilizers dictate whether you'd live or die. And now you wonder why you're sick? It can't get much clearer. God is saying to you, 'If you want to die, that's fine. But you'll have to do it my way.'"

Father P. left a short time later. I finished tearing up the flowers. Then I asked for a sleeping pill. Just one.

Our group includes representatives of many of the major religions in our country, along with members who describe themselves as "not affiliated with any religion." We recognize that living with MS has had a profound effect on our spiritual development, over and above any religious beliefs we may each hold. In view of that, I asked our ladies to share some thoughts about the impact of MS on their spiritual lives.

▲▲▲

PAT — Lynn, your idea for this topic surprised me just a little because about a year after my diagnosis, I wrote an article for a Christian magazine dealing with how MS has affected me, both physically and spiritually. I looked it over not too long ago to see how much my attitudes and feelings might have changed and grown over the years. I believe I have grown, but not necessarily because the MS caused it to happen.

When I was first diagnosed with MS, it came as a surprise to me only because I really didn't know much about it. The fact that something was wrong with me never shocked me; I never got upset, or questioned, or wondered, or had any of the feelings many go through. I automatically went to God for help. Now, I am not an overly religious person, but I do believe and my beliefs are strong. When this first started, I never asked the "why me?" question. I suppose I felt I had no reason to ask.

When my first major exacerbation hit and landed me in a wheelchair, I took it rather well. Or so I thought. But after a few months in a wheelchair, hassles and annoyances that I never knew existed came into play in a major way. Our house had stairs to the bedroom and bath that I could no longer access, and we could not afford to move. Then there were the trips to stores where the elevators were hidden, the restroom doors opened out or were too heavy to manage on my own, and the bathroom stalls wouldn't accommodate a wheelchair. The list goes on and on. And so annoyance and frustration entered my life with MS. But God never left my life and my beliefs never wavered. I don't believe that God caused my MS, that it was either a gift or a punishment from him.

My beliefs in God since becoming ill have only continued to grow and expand. I have found that MS in itself hasn't actually "given" me anything, but that I have sought out more things, more areas of exploration, because God has led me in that direction and I have chosen to follow.

I suppose I don't really believe MS is a good thing at all. It is an illness. A dreaded one. And I have it. That much I know. Whatever good comes from it comes from the fact that I have searched something out and found it waiting for me. God puts people, places, things in our paths. It is up to us whether we choose to meet that person, visit that place, look into that thing, stroll down that path. When something comes my way, I take a peek and see what's in store. If it looks promising, I follow, always hoping for the best. If it starts to feel not quite right, I'm out of there in a flash.

When others talk about what MS has given them, I can't seem to find one thing that I can say it has given me, except for its symptoms, the need for medications, the many doctor visits, the bad eyesight, the loss of my driving ability. Please do not think I mention these things as complaints, because that is not the case. I am merely stating what I do attribute to MS.

Am I different somehow? Am I missing something here? At first I did wonder about that. But not any longer. With all my being, I believe that MS is just one of those illnesses that has snuck into my life, with no invitation from me. But it is here now. For better or worse. The bad times come, the bad times go. The good times come, the good times go.

Multiple sclerosis has given me trials and troubles. God has provided a way around all of them. I try to watch for those ways and grasp at every one he provides. I might have missed some. In fact, I'm sure I have. But what I have found has given me more happiness than I'd ever imagined.

▲▲▲

JANE — Lynn, this is an area I'd like to contribute to. I know MS has dovetailed with my spiritual growth, because it's an area where I've changed so much in the twenty-four years since I've known about the MS.

Because MS hits us so essentially, it is a major push for our spiritual growth or stagnation. I think that at some point we all need to come to peace with the question, "Why has this happened to me?" I can't remember ever asking this, but I must have, and I implicitly answered it with, "Why *not* me?" Evil was introduced in the Garden, and it affects everyone, regardless of whether they're "deserving." As it turns out, my "evil," like that of so many others who have the diagnosis, is really not that bad. I believe God has wanted to use my essentially upbeat, positive experiences and nature to help others online and to provide balance and hope to many others. And that's why I spend so much time online facilitating support groups and operating in a leadership capacity. I have even been rewarded with beginning the GodandMS worship service for a Christian group; it has met weekly for the past eight months and it provides a deep measure of support to a group of approximately twenty regulars.

I have always drawn on the Lord to help me cope with the symptoms which I found difficult, and which I was essentially bearing alone. I regularly turn to God for help in dealing with the obnoxious, nebulous nature of MS itself. Prayer has become a daily, vital link, a means to cope with the inherent frustration of my hidden curse. I've also been redirected in my thinking and priorities to a higher spiritual realm where I find comfort, peace, and an expanded way of living that helps me cope with day-to-day life.

As my children grew, I began intensive bible study. Growth in my faith and the development of a living prayer relationship with God became priorities for me. I think these were so important to me because the MS was such a fundamental part of my life. I was implicitly looking for additional support as I sought a deeper kind of understanding.

Because I am dealing with an uncertain future, I turned long ago to my faith as ballast. God has been faithful and has provided everything I have needed at every turn. MS is a big-name disease and, because of the uncertainty and frustration accompanying it, I need the source of life and provider of every good gift right along with me in every step I take. I haven't settled for less, and I have been blessed, I think, especially in my attitude toward MS. I have that sorted through, and I bring to any situation a fundamentally positive view of what will be. I attribute my attitude to my faith in God and his care and protection of me, and to my gratitude for that care. I think whatever good befalls me comes from God, and that makes me even more open to additional good because my willingness to praise God in all circumstances affects who I am as a person.

I was able to find peace with my MS when I gave everything about me to God, when I allowed him to direct and control what happens to me in the future. I believe my faith grew just as my ability to surrender everything to God began to make sense to me, and as it began to be what I really want in life.

I had an MRI in January after not having had one for nine years. It actually showed lesions (spots/demyelinization) that were *less* bright and deep than before. That, of course, was unusual, and the only thing that had changed in those nine years was that I had made a concerted effort to deepen my spirituality and increase my bible study and my prayer relationship with God. I had taken my old MRI with me, and when the radiologist reviewed it after doing my new one, he came out to the hall to speak with me. He was impressed with the change. Before I left, he said, "Well, the good Lord sure is taking care of you." Right!

[GodandMS meets in the AOL private room (available through the People Connection) at 9:00 P.M. EST every Sunday, for one hour. The room accomodates approximately 22 people currently. Christians with MS (or their families) of any denomination are welcome. The meeting follows a worship format.]

▲▲▲

DEE — As you know, I was a hospital chaplain, which should mean that I was "religious." Although I certainly did my share of praying with people and for people, leading religious rites, etc., most of what I did was not religious in the sense most of us associate with that word. It was human spirituality or plain old human support, because you are a human being and so am I.

The worst thing that happened was when groups from certain churches would come in and "pray over" a person and "demand" that he/she be healed. It always left the person who had the illness feeling guilty and devastated. I can't tell you how many, many times that happened. It is bad theology, if one can call it that. It is plain wrong, in my opinion. My thoughts are: We are all humans with the frailties and vulnerabilities of being human and having a human body. Things happen to human bodies—God doesn't make things happen to people; he doesn't make them sick or disabled. Things happen because of our vulnerability to all sorts of illnesses, accidents, etc.

I believe it helps to pray, but it doesn't always result in healing. I came up with this idea when I was taking my training. I worked with leukemia patients a lot, and most of them were children. This constantly broke my heart. I watched how all the parents prayed their hearts out for their children to be healed. Some were healed and some weren't. What does that say to me? God picks and chooses? I don't think so! We don't know everything—I believe only God does. Others believe in another Higher Power or something that helps them sort out this mystery we call life. It all boils down to the fact that we are vulnerable and can't control everything.

▲▲▲

In some of these reflections, it's obvious that the writer belongs to a particular denomination. For instance, every aspect of my life was inexorably tied into and influenced by my lifelong membership in the Roman Catholic Church. I couldn't ignore that fact when I found my relationship with God changing, as it had to when the MonSter began to interrupt or intercept my every prayer. I still have to identify that connection when I reflect on the spiritual refinement that has taken place in my life over the past twenty-some years.

Others in our group, though, aren't specific about their religious ties. Some don't claim any religious belief beyond the tenet that we each carry within us a sustaining spirit.

▲▲▲

HELEN — I don't think my beliefs or lack thereof have had much effect on how I view my MS. I don't think the MS has either strengthened or weakened those beliefs I do have. I just try to live my life, as I would if I didn't have MS, in such a way that I won't have to come back the next time as a victim of oppression under Idi Amin. I honor the souls of *all* living beings, not just the human ones. That's where I find my spirituality, not in what some disease can do to me.

I do believe that some of my physical stuff is a carryover from problems I had in past lives. I hope I can work through them this time—it would be nice to leave the MonSter behind when I return again.

▲▲▲

JOY — Somebody here once said something about people with MS not loving Jesus enough and not wanting to get well.

This reminds me of an HBO documentary about hospice care. Did any of you happen to see it, several years ago? One of the terminally ill patients featured was a sweet little black woman whose pastor kept visiting her and promising her that if she had enough faith, she would be healed. So she never acknowledged, aloud at least, that she was dying. As a result, neither she nor her family members were able to get past denial and say proper goodbyes, and grieve normally. It was so sad that I wanted to kick some butt.

And then we could get into the metaphysical aspects of whether our Higher Selves choose our own destinies before birth for reasons our conscious human selves neither remember nor can comprehend. But that's another thing entirely. It isn't about guilt, or wishing ourselves well, or anything so superficial.

▲▲▲

I'm awed by these replies—so many of our members came up with summaries of their spiritual evolution right off the bat. Their philosophies might vary greatly. But every members seems to be able to say, in her own words, "Okay, this is what I believe, this is what I don't believe, I know these things for sure. Now let's keep that in mind and get on with life." They downplay the roller-coaster rides they might have endured on the way to their conclusions.

Renee opted to share some of her "ride" with us:

▲▲▲

Marla and I went shopping one Saturday afternoon recently, and I found this really great little sexy black dress. Very unlike me, but this dress was awesome, reasonably priced, fit like a dream, and was made by one of those designers who lie so that when it says you are wearing a size three, it's probably actually the equivalent of a size seven.

To make things better, my hubby's old girlfriend was behind the counter when we checked out. She used to brag to me at every opportunity about all the stuff she and my hubby used to do for fun. But there she was, and she had gained approximately seventy pounds and cut her hair, which on her just doesn't work. So now I was really on a roll, because I'm tiny, I've got the long blond hair (so what if it's a wig?) and the short black dress, and Burt and I were going out on a Saturday night.

After Marla left, I met Burt at his office, and he started to follow me home. I had the radio on full blast, listening to some of my favorite songs from back around 1979–80. I was remembering that back then I could do anything and everything I wanted, I had the energy of a million wild horses, I loved life, my kids, my job, everything.

And I started to cry. Driving down the road, I started to cry so hard it took my breath away. And for the first time in my life, I yelled, "I hate you, God! For MS, for taking all those years away, and for all the things I can't do anymore, I hate you!" I had never felt so alone, so empty, so hopeless, and so tired in my whole life. Here I had been planning this night out, and I realized I already was too tired to even drive home, much less to go out anywhere.

I'm only forty-five years old. I realized that I'm tired of being tired all the time. Tired of not being able to remember stuff. Tired of not being able to pee when I need to. Tired of not being able to tell if I went to the bathroom on myself, because I am so numb everywhere.

For the first time since the first two years after I was diagnosed, I was scared. I realized I had never really said all this stuff to anyone, because they might have gotten scared about how badly I was really doing or thought I was feeling sorry for myself. And I would rather die than be pitied. Staying in the problem never, ever got me into the solution, so I'd always tended to look for the bright side.

But this time there just wasn't a bright side. So I cried. Burt, following me home, apparently figured out that I was really upset, because he signaled me to pull over at the grocery store. He asked me what was wrong, and I let it all out. How I am tired of trying to be fine when I'm really not. How I am tired all the time. Period. How I am worse, and how I'm getting still worse. How I worry about how that affects him and Dominic (my grandson, whom we're raising).

Am I still in the anger/grief stage of acceptance? Who knows? All I know is that I feel this loneliness that I have never felt in my whole life. Because no one can help me come to grips with how this disease has progressed, except for me and God. Not Burt, not my therapist. And God (whom I love dearly and talk to on a regular basis) isn't working fast enough for me. I know he is listening. I know he cares for me and loves me. But is there a lesson I'm supposed to be learning here?

See, I used to be able to pull myself up by my bootstraps, put on my smiley face, make jokes, and just do whatever needed to be done. But the truth is that the bootstraps broke. The smiley face is now transparent (you should see the dark circles under my eyes). There is no peace, no rest from this disease anymore. I am tired, not just of the MS fatigue, but tired of everything.

When we got home that day, I decided to just give up. I lay down on my bed, crying (gee, I have been doing a lot of that lately) and praying as earnestly as I have ever prayed, asking especially for awareness of a sign that God is working in all our lives. I found myself finally saying that if this is the way my life is going to be, I give up. I quit. I cannot do this. I gave it my best shot. I want to die. Right now.

So, okay, I closed my eyes to see if there was a sign in those little squiggles you see when you close your eyes. Nothing I could make sense of.

Burt came in and I cried and prayed for awareness, the whole nine yards. Little by little, I sobbed out what I was truly feeling; to hell with whether he could handle it or not. That is his problem. I told him I feel that MS is slowly eating away my heart and soul.

Well, needless to say, I eventually got better. A little better, anyway. That pissed me off. I looked at the ceiling and said, "What? I have to just get up and keep going? Is that it? That's it?" And that was it.

I'm still scared. Scared absolutely to death. Scared because for the first time I have zero control in all areas, because nothing works.

At the same time, I trust that God has a plan and that eventually it will all work out. But what do you do with the pain and fear (other than ask him to remove it) while you are waiting for it all to work out? When everything you once did to cope no longer works? This is a first for me.

I've prayed that the loneliness would go away. So come on, God, whatever the reason is, let's get started. Limboland has never appealed to me. Where is this disease truly going (never mind the B.S. the doctors used to tell me—that it won't get worse, blah, blah, blah)?

I go back to God again and again. I pray for awareness of signs that he is working in my life. Eventually I will get them.

▲▲▲

TARA — Before I knew I had MS, and before it slowed me down a bit, I thought that I as an individual had to "save the world." I didn't see the interconnectedness of the world. I was very hyper and running between this and that project and always zooming along until I crashed. I like to compare my life then to a whirling dervish. I went like crazy, but even if I was aiming in one direction, I had a hard time getting there because I was zipping all over the place in circles and only stopped to examine what I was doing with my life when I ran out of energy and toppled over onto my side. I always worked independently and couldn't see the things around me at all, at least not until I ran smack into them!

Then the MS got to where I had to roll along more slowly, and I found myself lying on my side (so to speak) more often. Of course, that made me look more closely at what was right there beside me. I realized that if I could offer anything to the world, I would have to do it on a team level. In other words, I found out that I was only the center of my own universe, not of everybody's. I think the most profound enlightenment that I have had since the MS has progressed is that the best thing that I can offer to my fellow earth dwellers is unconditional love. It's such a simple thing, yet I don't think I really even knew what it was when I was younger.

I found that if I was to make a difference in the world, it was going to happen in the little things that I did and said for others. I feel now that I do make a difference, because I have joined the communal spirit of all around me and about me. If I offer a bit of myself that can bring a smile to someone else, they in turn will pass it on. If one person is a little kinder and gentler because of the love that I offer, that is a huge accomplishment.

I never would have seen the simplicity of life had I not had the guidance of a Higher Power to speak to me in those moments that the MS gifted to me.

Well, I guess you can tell that, although the MS brings

many challenges, it also has brought me a huge gift, and for
that I am eternally grateful.

▲▲▲

JAMIE — Very well said, Tara. I also think of my MS as a gift
in many ways. Had I not been dealt the MS, I may have never
learned gratitude for what I'm able to do. And I might not have
learned what life is really about, which is love, tolerance, and
helping others.

▲▲▲

We're back to Father P. now. Which is where I had to return all
those years ago, as soon as the sleeping pill wore off. I knew intel-
lectually, even then, that he'd been spouting a bunch of baloney.
But some small part of me, the part that had been overeducated in
the "fear God and/or be punished" theory, accepted it as valid.
After all, I had left the convent, tried to commit suicide, lots of
other horrible stuff. Hadn't I? I'd known, even before I made my
choices, that they might be the wrong ones. Hadn't I? So what
more (or less) could I expect than to be justly penalized by a sen-
tence of life with the MonSter?

Looking back, I see that I let Father P.'s words be the operative
force in my life for the next twenty years. In some silent way, there
at the beginning, I promised God that I'd work for him as long as
he wanted me to, meaning as long as he kept the MS away so I
could work. And I promised myself that as long as I continued in
that way, hidden within the confines of the Church, the MS would
leave me alone. I got completely wrapped up in this commitment,
almost to the point of ignoring Ron and my girls. My daytime jobs
were with the church or with agencies of the church. My evenings
and weekends were spent volunteering for just about any church
committee that would have me. Even my social life revolved primarily around priests, nuns, and other "churchy" people. I blamed
any unrest that I felt in my soul during those years on my own

inability to recognize and accept the peace that God was surely willing to offer me.

Of course, in spite of my defense strategy, the disease progressed. Eventually I couldn't work anymore, couldn't keep pace with all my church-based associations, couldn't even get to church or, if I did manage to get there, couldn't sit through a service. I felt rejected by God, kicked off his team, thrown out of his house. He wasn't willing to bargain with me any longer.

I had to admit to myself that I no longer believed in God, not the God of fear and punishment who I'd been taught about all my life. Not the God who would punish me for having an emotional illness by giving me a serious physical illness. Not the God who would penalize me for following my heart by making sure that I wasn't able to "follow" anything ever again.

Ironically, I think it was at this point that I finally began to experience something of a close, personal relationship with God. Isolated for the most part from communal spiritual endeavors, I was somehow freed to head out on my own to find peace with my Higher Power and his works in my life. Since then, I've spent a lot of time reading, talking, listening, and praying about this. Over the past five or six years, I've come to see that God is too big to be categorized or interpreted or understood by any of the limited means available to us humans. There is simply no way to accurately second-guess God or his intentions.

At the same time, I've experienced God in many clearly defined aspects that both expanded and refined my perception of him. Looking back, I recognize that, while my spin into potential spiritual oblivion was effected in large part by a priest, one of the threads that kept me grounded as a spiritual being was another priest. During those years of immersing myself in church life, I worked with and became close friends with Father C. His tenacious hold on me as a human being worth "saving" was indeed the major factor in my salvation (I'm not necessarily referring only to the state of my immortal soul here). While I've only seen him a few times in the past fifteen or so years (he has been working as a missionary in Africa), his friendship with Ron and me, and his influence on our lives has always been a sort of anchor in my faith. I don't think I've evolved in my faith exactly as Father C. might have planned. Still, I've been validated every step of the way by what he taught me and still teaches me in our long-distance communications.

On my own, I can review my Catholic catechism now, and I can honestly agree with much of what is there. I can do this not because any "authority" on such matters tells me that my agreement is mandatory, but because I can see "my" God's hand in whatever truth is proclaimed in the catechism. I can say, "Yes, I believe that I'm made in the image and likeness of God." Then I'm free to go beyond that and say what I really feel my belief entails: "This means that I and every other living being, as his creatures, share something of God, some part of his life force. We are an immeasurable measure of the same infinite, creative, loving energy that he is. As a God-image, my mission is to share that energy with others, as he has shown us how to do." I believe absolutely that God will always be less concerned with how many rules we've blindly followed or how much doctrine we've memorized than with how much of our "Godness" we've managed to share with others.

At that point, I stop and wonder. As a God-image, I wouldn't want to inflict something like multiple sclerosis on any other living being. How can I imagine (even after being told!) that God himself could be less merciful than I am? God (or whatever we choose to name our Higher Power) can do nothing but good. If this Higher Power had anything at all to do with my MS, it can only be that I'm supposed to effect some good by having it.

So I'm sorry, Father P. You're wrong. *Dead* wrong. Maybe I'll never know exactly what I'm supposed to accomplish by having multiple sclerosis. But I know for sure that it will be something good, some way of sharing God's life force with someone else. It is not a punishment for being human.

16

Purple Legs
and Dancing Faces

We hear it so often, even from professionals who are highly skilled in the care of people with multiple sclerosis: "[Insert weird sign or symptom here] has nothing to do with MS." But mention that same weird sign or symptom to a group of people who live with MS and hands will shoot up, with shouts of "Me, too! Me, too!" coming from all over the room. It can be some minor, quirky thing, hardly worth our attention. Or it can be something so bizarre that it's almost impossible to believe that more than one person can end up with the same thing.

Purple legs, for instance. One evening last year, Karen mentioned to me that my legs looked funny. They did look and feel kind of puffy, but I didn't think much of it. The only time I'd ever had that problem previously was when I was pregnant. I knew I wasn't pregnant this time, and I had too much else on my mind to look for the cause. We had spent the day at my brother's funeral, so I dismissed it as the result of standing for so long at the funeral home and the cemetery.

That night, though, when I took off the black stockings I'd been wearing, I saw that, besides being swollen, my legs had bright-purple squiggles running in clusters from ankle to groin. I managed to push that little bit of information out of my actively conscious mind for the next few days, until Julie said to me, "Mom, your legs look like Grandma's." I didn't know if she was referring to my mother or Ron's, but either way, it wasn't a compliment.

Several weeks later, at my next appointment with Dr. C., my primary-care physician, I showed him my legs. He gave me a prescription for a diuretic, which eased the swelling but did nothing for the discoloration. Within the next few weeks, my arms decided to get in on the act, too, taking on a somewhat lighter mauve mottling. At that point, Dr. C. referred me to a vascular surgeon. That freaked me out a little bit—I imagined that Dr. C. thought that something was horribly wrong, maybe a blockage in a major artery, which would cause all my limbs to shrivel up and fall off.

The vascular guy ran some simple tests to measure circulation, then propped my legs up and pressed on one of them in a toe-to-top sweeping motion. The purple disappeared.

He assured me that there was no real danger. He said that the problem was neurological in origin, that the blood vessels in my extremities weren't getting the message from the brain telling them to contract and expand in order to push the blood through.

I asked, "You mean it's caused by the MS?"

He said that, in essence, that's exactly what caused it. Major shock! This guy, a bona fide doctor, didn't intend to test me for every possible disorder of the circulatory system. He wasn't going to try to make me believe that MS could not be responsible for something beyond what had already been printed in the medical textbooks!

He recommended walking, massage, and support stockings, along with diuretics when the swelling was bothersome. It's true that some of these remedies aren't so easy to incorporate into my daily life (I'm supposed to walk for exercise when my legs don't work? Do all the times that I have to "run" to the bathroom after taking the diuretic count as exercise?). I have managed, though, to keep the swelling down on a somewhat consistent basis, and I just wear long clothes to cover my colorful legs and arms. But I'd finally found a doctor who was willing to look at the full scope of MS's effects, over and above all the "sanctioned" ones.

Relieved as I was at his diagnosis, this was the first time I'd ever heard of swelling or discoloration of the extremities associated with MS. I thought that I was the ultimate oddball! But when I mentioned the purple legs to others in the Froup, I got a flurry of replies saying, "Hey, that's happened to me, too!"

I've also read that discoloration of the extremities can be caused by Amantadine, a prescription medication used by some people to treat MS-related fatigue. But not all of us who have purple legs are also taking Amantadine, and some who take the drug don't have purple legs. The only thing we all have in common is MS.

Another weird symptom that comes up often in our conversations is an odd kind of "internal trembling" to which we all seem susceptible:

▲▲▲

RENEE — Does anyone have the inside shaking? I have that once in a while, and until it comes out and develops into real tremors, I can't stand it. It feels like something terrifying is going to happen, or it's a nervous thing, or. . . . I can't describe the feeling, really. It goes away after the shaking starts on the outside.

▲▲▲

That's exactly what I have, almost every evening. It's one of the most uncomfortable things that I've ever experienced. It usually happens while I'm just trying to sit and unwind after a busy day. I feel like my insides (not just my innards, like my stomach and attached organs, but everything inside my skin, all the way to fingertips and toes) are "nervous." It's kind of like every part of my body is about to go into its own private panic attack. No part of me is willing or able to just sit still. It's like I have restless leg syndrome in my whole body. I remind myself of a dog straining at the leash. The only thing that seems to help is putting my feet up on Ron's lap and having him rub them *hard!* I guess that gives me a place to focus all that "sensory energy" that's accumulated to the point of overflowing.

▲▲▲

JOY — When I read Renee's note, I wondered if I've experienced what she describes or something that's not quite the same. My tremors have never moved on to exterior shaking or spasms. But Lynn, what I often have sounds a lot like what you are talking about. For years I thought I was having mild anxiety attacks or panic attacks, which later turned out to be associated with MS (according to what others have told me).

▲▲▲

LORI — That is one of my worst symptoms. I have that practically all the time, and if I overdo it, it gets even worse. The outside shaking gets worse, too. God forbid I should be trying to do something delicate—like, oh, taking a drink, maybe?—when that thing happens. Gets kind of messy!

▲▲▲

DONNA — It's not fun having the shakes. I shake externally when I wake up in the morning, and I have learned to be extremely cautious with coffee and cigarettes for the first thirty minutes or so after getting up. Try to remember that this, too, shall pass; if it doesn't, you won't need a mixer to make instant pudding!

The internal shakes, though, are more difficult to deal with. I try to stay busy and keep my mind occupied to distract myself from the discomfort. It is not painful, but it feels as though all of my body is full of too much energy and is trying to dissipate the energy through the vibrations.

I compare it with the "fight or flight" syndrome that occurs during and after a traumatic event. Adrenaline rushes through your body in order to give you the strength to run away from or fight the threat. When the threat is removed, it takes time for the adrenaline level to return to normal, and sometimes your (my) body shakes as that level drops.

I talked with my neurologist about it. His only suggestions were to avoid excess stimulation and to distract myself while it is going on. *Duh!* I suggested he get one of those long vibrators, turn it on high, swallow it, and then tell me about distracting myself. He asked if I ever thought I might be just a little twisted. I replied, "I'm fine, but I'm still shaking!" Fortunately, he appreciates sarcasm. So do I.

▲▲▲

Another idiosyncrasy that most of us can claim is Wal-Mart Syndrome. This isn't necessarily restricted to Wal-Mart or even to department stores in general; it can occur in any place where there are too many external stimuli to process at once, where our senses are bombarded to the point of dangerous overload. Wal-Mart is the scapegoat only because we've all had this experience in similar large, busy, colorful establishments. When we walk into a bustling, crowded area, we aren't only aware of people moving among racks of clothes (or desks or theater seats or restaurant tables), with the sounds of conversations and public announcements and tinkling silverware in the background. We see a tangled, moving mass of colors and forms, and we hear a chaotic jumble of noises, all waiting to assault us if we blink or cough or scratch our heads or do anything other than focus on our destinations and walk or wheel ourselves straight to the desired spot. If we linger too long once we get there, the bedlam catches up, and we find that we can no longer remember how to talk or move or even breathe.

▲▲▲

HELEN — Wal-Mart Syndrome, as I define it, is being in any place or situation that puts me into overload, whether it's an overload of visual stimulation, sound/noise, movement, colors, or anything that is just too much. It goes right through my head and causes me mental, physical, and emotional pain, confusion, dizziness, disorientation, the whole nine yards. I have to seek out quieter malls than I used to, and I know I won't be going to Summerfest this year. I hope I can make it for Indian Summer Festival and Irish Fest, both of which I go to for the food and the music.

I don't know how I can do these things yet keep out of overload mode. If anybody has any suggestions, I would be ever so grateful. This scares me more than almost any other of my myriad symptoms, because it's so out of my control. I have fibromyalgia, too, and this problem is common in both MS and fibro, so I suppose I have a double helping of it.

Oh well, just send me food, soda, and purple Gak, and I will hole up in my new bed with some Irish tapes.

▲▲▲

DEE — I have been troubled by fluorescent lighting and movement in malls, patterns in rugs, etc. I always get an aura and double vision first. I may have mentioned this before, but the first time this happened I was about eighteen, had just gotten married, and was sweeping a braided rug with a broom (because we couldn't afford a vacuum cleaner). All of a sudden I couldn't see; everything was moving. My then-husband and I used to call it "shaky eyes."

Well, my hubby and I went to a new restaurant the other night and I knew immediately that I was going to have trouble—it was very bright and noisy, with lots of people, lots of activity. We'd just sat down when I began having double vision, "shaky eyes," and flashes of light. It was bad, but I was hoping it would go away, and besides, I did not want to disappoint Al, as we had not been anywhere in quite a while.

So, he read me the menu; I could not see it at all. We ordered, and in about twenty minutes or so it began to go away, but replacing it was something like a knife going through my left eye. It was very painful and I was really dizzy. As soon as we finished eating, we rushed home and I went to bed. In two or three hours, it was gone. It was one of the worst spells I've had, but then I think I always say that.

It's simply the pits, having to disappoint family, especially because of illness—I really hate that.

Then we have dancing faces. . . .

▲▲▲

ME — I swear this is happening. I am having these muscle spasms today, bad ones, on the left side of my nose! Honest, this is really going on. I have to go to the store soon, but I started thinking about the sight I would make at the counter with my face dancing all around. Just the left side.

I wouldn't tell this to anyone but you guys. Nobody else would believe me.

▲▲▲

RENEE — Can you please get someone to videotape this phenomenon—I have never seen a dancing face. Does it hurt?

▲▲▲

ME — It doesn't hurt. It's just a plain old spaz, but it picked a strange spot to show up. I also get bugs crawling in my ears and through my brains (or at least it feels like that). I tried to tell one of my doctors about it and he gave me his pat answer: "Hmm, that's interesting."

▲▲▲

JAMIE — Hey! I get that too! It's like ants or something marching in my brain. I can even "hear" the sort of crunching noise they make. I told my doctor I had "cola" headaches—you know, it feels like when you swim and get water up your nose, that fizzy feeling in the back of the head.

▲▲▲

Most people don't pick up conversations in the hum of air conditioners, fans, computer equipment, clothes dryers, or whatever. We do. Many of us are able to "hear voices" in what's supposed to be white noise. We can't understand exactly what's being said, but it's definitely a dialogue rather than just one person speaking. Maybe our household appliances (or our ears?) are tuned into a low-volume broadcast of *The Twilight Zone*.

▲▲▲

HELEN — I used to "hear" what sounded like radio conversations real softly in the background of whatever noise was within earshot. I thought it was some kind of strange ESP thing. Never did figure out what it really was. Now I can't even remember when it happened.

▲▲▲

Other Froup members report seeing people talk (up close!) but being unable to hear them. Some say that their own voices sound like they're disconnected, that they're coming from other people in other places. They say, too, that even "real" noises can have unexpected, exaggerated effects.

▲▲▲

DONNA — Noises in general have been getting to me. The phone ringing sends electricity all over my body. The squeals of the grandkids send me running (shuffling) to another room for some quiet time. It's really hard to explain it to someone who doesn't "feel" sounds. I've offered to hook the adult members of my family up to the appliance of their choice and then shock them occasionally to let them see how it feels. They all said they would take my word for it. I guess they aren't as electrically inclined as I am.

▲▲▲

This is another quirk that I have major trouble with, too. Ebby, my best-buddy dog for the past twelve years, has one fault. He's a barker. Lately, for the past year or so, his bark grates on all my nerves. I've thought about using ear plugs, but the irritation doesn't seem in any way connected to my ears, although they transmit the "shocks" to my brain and spine. It actually hurts! Then I get p.o.d at myself because I end up having such mean thoughts about an innocent dog!

▲▲▲

HELEN — I was thinking (oh, the strain!) about the fact that so many of us have problems with overloaded sensory input. Maybe that's why having this group is so good—we can talk all we want, and we don't have to do it where it's noisy or crowded. If we did all get together in person, at least we'd understand if one of us asked to be excused and went outdoors for a while. It's a real bitch to explain to someone who doesn't have the problem, isn't it? I mean, here I am, nearly deaf in my right ear, and still so sensitive to sound that I'm tempted to start wearing ear plugs twenty-four hours a day, seven days a week.

▲▲▲

How about normally abnormal body temperatures? I was surprised when I found out that this is a characteristic many of us share. My own body temperature has always been lower than normal. The obstetrician I saw when I was expecting Karen routinely diagnosed pregnancies before a physical examination by having the patient track her basal (first-thing-in-the-morning) temperatures. Those were supposed to be low, in the normal, nonpregnant woman. But if they were elevated from 97.-something to 98.-something during certain days of her cycle, then the woman was probably pregnant. My basal temperature, however, never went above 97.5 degrees. So Dr. T. told me I couldn't be pregnant. I insisted that I was, and I made an appointment for an examination. I was pregnant.

Thereafter, I'd get frustrated every time I came down with a cold or the flu or something else that made me feel feverish. I'd call the doctor and the receptionist would ask, "Do you have a fever?"

I'd say something like, "Well, the thermometer says I don't, but I feel hot and achy, so I think I do."

And the receptionist would say, "If you don't have a fever, you probably don't need treatment." So I'd end up literally sweating it out, whatever it was, on my own.

Some years after I was diagnosed with multiple sclerosis, I heard or read that people who have MS are very heat intolerant, that anything that increases body temperature (fevers, saunas or hot baths, even eating a bowl of hot soup) can exacerbate MS symptoms, at least temporarily. I knew that was true from my own experience. But it never occurred to me to ascribe my normally abnormal temperature to MS.

Then I got to know my cyber-buddies, and the subject came up several times.

▲▲▲

LORI — Seems I decided to go out and catch myself strep throat with a double ear infection. Whoopee! I feel like I've been run over by a truck. The thing that drives me nuts is that most doctors, when they take my temperature, tell me that I don't have a fever. They don't believe that my normal temperature is around 96.8 or 97.1 degrees, so if I get up around 99 or 100 degrees, I'm pretty miserable and so achy that I can barely move. How about you guys? I have heard that it is common for MSers to have rather low normal temps. I'm always cold, and sometimes my hands get so cold that they turn white and stiff and my nailbeds turn purple. It doesn't matter if it's 32 degrees or 102 degrees out; my hands still do this. My arms and legs are perfectly warm and toasty—no problems there. On rare occasions my feet get cold, but nothing like my hands.

▲▲▲

RENEE — Lori, that sounds just like me. Fortunately, my primary-care doctor knows this and adjusts his thinking accordingly. I am really sorry you are sick. I've had strep throat and ear infections, but not both at once. Awful. In fact, I have never heard of anyone getting both ears and strep all at once. My, my, a major coup! *Not!* Rest and drink liquids (you know all this— you're a mom, for heaven's sake). Just take it easy. Let everybody wait on you for a change.

▲▲▲

JAMIE — Lori, so sorry you are sick. I hope you feel better soon. I, too, have low normal temperatures and cold hands. Some of my friends say they are going to buy me gloves because my hands are so cold, even in summer! When I'm hot, I'm hot all over, and the same with cold. Usually my "thermostat" is the opposite of everyone else's. If they are hot, I'm cold, and if they are cold, I'm hot!

▲▲▲

Here's a real biggie: the can't-swallow-choke-a-lot syndrome. This is something that is now recognized as a real MS effect. I've even seen references to it in medical literature, and most of our doctors seem to take it seriously when we complain about it. The only thing we dispute is the claim, in published material and by most of our doctors, that this is something that shows up only in the more advanced cases of MS. Many in our group have had only minor symptoms so far, but they still have major trouble swallowing.

I've had this problem for several years, since before I had any suspicion that I was an "advanced case." It has been mostly just an annoying aspect of life with MS. But on occasion it can be potentially dangerous. Recently, for instance, I got a vitamin C tablet caught in my throat. I couldn't get it down, and my gag and choke reflexes were so weak that they were ineffective in bringing it back up. So it just sat there in my throat. By the time it melted, my throat felt burned, as though I'd swallowed some kind of caustic liquid. That feeling persisted for several days, until I ended up with a wracking, hacking cough, one that produced nothing but a lot of noise and more coughing. When I called Dr. C. about it, he wanted me to go for x-rays. But I didn't have transportation at the time, so he ordered an antibiotic instead, and the condition cleared up with no further problems.

This incident did teach me to be very careful when trying to ingest anything that's too big to swallow easily. Even that precaution isn't entirely foolproof, since the difficulty can occur at just about any time, with even the smallest bits of food refusing to go down.

I heard one doctor say that this is all probably caused by some of the medications prescribed for MS people, which can cause dryness of the mouth. I have a question about the validity of that observation, though, because every one of us has reported that clear liquids are one of the hardest things to swallow. Why is that, if the problem is caused by dryness of the mouth? I talked with Dr. R.'s assistant about the swallowing trouble; she actually told me to avoid clear liquids when it's acting up. I wonder how we're supposed to avoid our own saliva?

RENEE — Lynn, about swallowing problems and not drinking liquids: that is a catch-22 for me because if I don't drink liquids, I get dehydrated very, very fast, and I get kidney and/or bladder infections. I hate that you have the swallowing problem, but I am glad someone knows what I am talking about when I describe it. I, too, have gotten pills stuck in my throat. And I couldn't get them up or down, and they actually kind of quickly dissolved, which tasted awful and irritated my throat for a few days. Why can't pills be made smaller? The sicker I get, the bigger the pills, it seems.

▲▲▲

KIM — A speech therapist I work with deals with this problem all the time in her practice. When I told her about it, she said, "Hmm. . . . That's not a good thing." I also find myself coughing on liquids a lot more than I used to. But I have the strongest cough this side of the Mason-Dixon line! So I generally don't get infections from aspirating fluids. I haven't even mentioned this to my doctor. Maybe I should?

▲▲▲

JANE — A computer friend told me to hum when I choke. This helps, but I'm not sure whether it is because it really works or because it makes me laugh instead! Do warn your family before you try this. My kids don't seem to care when I choke, but, boy, you should have heard them when I was both choking and humming!

▲▲▲

JANIS — Well, I know that when I have problems swallowing, it feels like the "system" just shuts off. Like the brain suddenly can't reach the throat and tell it what to do. It is scary to be sitting with a bite of food half down your throat but not going anywhere, just sitting there because the brain forgot to tell the throat how to work the food down! It's like having a lump in my throat, and I feel as if my throat is trying to get something down, but it's too tired to manage it. It doesn't hurt; it's just frightening. I haven't had it too often, thank goodness. But I've had it often enough to understand how scary it is. And I thought severe asthma was scary, when I couldn't breathe. This comes close.

▲▲▲

LORI — I've got a couple of questions. I heard you guys (notice how I said "heard," oh boy!) talking about choking on your own saliva. I do that quite frequently; as a matter of fact, the standard family joke is that they're going to have to call 911 for me. Try explaining that one! Is that part of the swallowing thing? Also, it seems to me that I swallow like I have a sore throat or something. You know, like my throat is swollen and it is difficult. Is that part of it, too?

▲▲▲

ME — It must be, Lori. I've actually been tempted sometimes to do something like the Heimlich maneuver on myself, but higher up. The food isn't way down where it obstructs breathing; it's just stuck in some kind of esophageal never-never land. It's uncomfortable but not enough of an acute irritant to cause the body to react reflexively to eject it. I keep thinking that if I could manage a good shove to the area right below my throat, I could get the stuff to pop out.

▲▲▲

As we got to know one another better, we discovered that we had many more things in common besides the medical or "problematic" things we've mentioned so far. We're talking about more basic commonalities, such as hair color, eye color, ancestry, etc. The ladies in the Froup decided to pursue this more carefully (albeit unscientifically) through a poll that asked each member a number of questions about herself.

Here are some of our findings:

— As children or young adults, we (meaning a large percentage of us) demonstrated a number of "differences" that were explained away as clumsiness or poor coordination, or were blamed on nerves or stress, for many years.

— We brought home report cards saying something to the effect of "Very intelligent, but doesn't apply herself." [HELEN — It's striking that we all seem to have started out with pretty high I.Q.s. Not that it has any bearing on our various ailments. It's just that we seem to be "birds of a feather" in more than a few ways.]

— We've had problems from childhood with mislaying things, forgetting to do homework, etc.

— We had problems doing things like speaking in class; even so many years ago, we had trouble getting our brains and mouths to work together.

— It was hard for us to be involved in projects that demanded attention from anybody outside our own group of "comfortable" people. As a result, many of us were perceived as being cliquish.

— We share an almost uncanny number of physical characteristics. Many of us have light or reddish hair, fair skin, and light or hazel eyes. On this common trait—light eyes—there's more evidence than what we gathered from our informal questionnaire. Dr. M., my first neurologist, said that almost all African-American MS patients have yellow or hazel flecks in their irises. [HELEN — It's known that people in temperate climates get MS, that it doesn't exist in tropical areas. I've known a lot of African-Americans that have it, but all were born in this country. Their ancestry may be mixed, giving them some of the same genes that whites have.]

— Members who are of Scots-Irish or other Northern European ancestry are in the majority. Again, there's documentation to support this—recent studies have pointed up a disproportionate number of Scots, in particular, in the MS population.

— Many of us were diagnosed with or suspected of having a learning problem that "disordered," displaced, or reversed the images we looked at. These diagnoses occurred even before dyslexia was recognized as a real medical condition. [HELEN — I could not, and still can't always, distinguish left from right. I could never comfortably do fine work, such as hand sewing, embroidery, etc. I once was assessed for vocational training. The counselor looked at my test scores and deadpanned, "You could probably do whatever you wanted to do. But I would seriously suggest that you never become a Swiss watch maker."]

— Virtually all of us were diagnosed during adulthood with lupus, rheumatoid arthritis, fibromyalgia, Crohn's disease, or other autoimmune/connective-tissue disorders. Symptoms of these were, for the majority of us, present even during our childhoods.

— We saw other medical similarities, in addition to the ones already discussed here. Many of us had sun sensitivity, migraines, and irritable bowel problems while growing up.

We've come up with a few hypotheses (or at least potential ones) from our research:

— We wonder if MS, rather than a nervous system disorder that eventually affects the brain, is actually a brain defect or disorder that manifests in early youth and progresses to more and more severe nervous system involvement over time.

— We wonder if there is a stronger familial predisposition toward MS than was previously suspected. Is it possible to assess a person as being at high risk for MS based only on careful scrutiny of that person's genetic history? This history would take into account genetic factors (like the light hair and eye colors) that are not now officially recognized as connected to MS. The history wouldn't even have to consider ancestors who had or may have had multiple sclerosis, although that would increase the risk even more.

— Is it possible that the genetic material that programs an embryo to develop seemingly inconsequential physical characteristics (such as amber flecks in the iris) may also program that embryo to develop multiple sclerosis twenty or thirty years down the road?

— It has been theorized that the place where a person spends the first fifteen years of his/her life plays a part in determining susceptibility to multiple sclerosis. For example, multiple sclerosis is very common in the Midwest of the United States; it's almost unheard of among African natives. But if a person lives in Indiana from birth to age fifteen and then moves to Kenya, his/her chance of getting MS won't be reduced. By the same token, a person who moves from Kenya to Indiana at the age of fifteen will probably never have MS. Is it possible that geography itself is a more significant risk factor than is currently recognized or suspected? And if so, does that geographical link apply only to the first fifteen years of a person's life or does it also hold true for the geographical heritages of one's parents, grandparents, etcetera?

— We wonder if researchers should concentrate more on tracing genetic traits than on tracking a virus as a causative agent in MS.

It would be nice (helpful? interesting? explosive?) if we could somehow pull all this information together and do something useful with it. Maybe we could find a way to trace MS back to its original source in each individual, starting with ancestors' area of birth and color of hair, or the number of warts on our grandmothers' chins. Maybe from that would come a way to prevent the disease. Maybe from that would come a way to cure the disease in those of us who already have it.

We can dream, can't we? In the meantime, it's at least fun to compare notes and find out that the weird things that aren't supposed to have anything to do with MS are common to all of us.

17

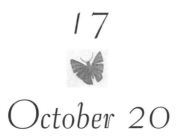

October 20

LORI — Geez, you guys. I have been in such a pissy mood. I'm sorry I've been in such a snit lately. I was feeling pretty good, so I basically ignored the fact that there is something wrong with me, and I set myself up for something. I'm not sure what.

On Saturday I decided to go walking around in 90-degree heat at a craft show for two hours (sans cane—thank God that Steve was there). I thought that if I just ignored the MS, it would go away. Well, dammit all, it didn't, and it's hitting me too hard to try to dismiss it.

I would like my life to be like that of other twenty-eight-year-olds. I'm tired of acting and feeling like an old lady. Is there nothing we can do to make this go away?

I guess I go through those times, like the rest of you, I'm sure, when I wonder whether I have "anything," and I think maybe I'm just lazy and getting older. But dammit, this isn't right. I am not lazy and I should *not* be feeling this way.

Don't get me wrong; I am far from suicidal. But don't you guys just wish it would all be over sometimes? Not in the morbid sense, but just so you wouldn't have to do this anymore? I am tired of hurting. I am tired of shaking. I am tired of being so weak that I can barely stand. I am tired of not being able to do things for and with Amanda. I am tired of falling on my ass. I am tired of having to use a freakin' cane. I am tired of my eyes not working, and of hurting all the time. I am tired of not being the kind of wife I should be because I feel like shit. I am tired of not being able to think of things I'm thankful for because I'm so friggin' busy being pissed off at the world and life in general.

I want to go hiking and rappelling like I used to. I want to run around like a maniac and not give a second thought to the energies I'm wasting. I want to send myself into total burnout. I want to be a part of a board meeting and make decisions that have impact.

I am so damned tired of being so damned useless. It took everything I had just to put the freakin' dishes in the dishwasher and do a load of laundry. And I had to do these things because I was too wiped out to do them over the weekend. So today, just when the fatigue peaked, I was faced with three or four days' worth of dishes and a week's worth of laundry.

I'm sorry I'm whining. I've been doing a lot of that lately. It just seems that things have been getting progressively worse since March. This is definitely my worst year. I was feeling so good there for a while, so I guess I just pushed it. I suppose it's my own fault, but I don't think I should be punished for wanting and trying to live a normal life. I am just tired. Sorry for dumping and being so depressing. Just one of those days, I guess. If you've gotten this far, thanks for coming along for the ride.

▲▲▲

Multiple sclerosis is a big disease. As we try to find ways of making our lives as MSers more liveable, we often shift our focus away from the immensity of the disease and its potential effects. We have to concentrate more on the small, troublesome realities of living with MS and deal with them one at a time, as each arises. If we find we can't drink from a glass without dropping and shattering it on the kitchen floor, we don't die of thirst; we buy some plastic tumblers. If we find we can't run three miles, we don't cut off our legs and hang ourselves on the back of the sofa; we grab a cane and walk a block. Or thirty steps. Or ten feet. It's manageable this way. The big, scary truth, the overwhelming, all-encompassing admission that "I have multiple sclerosis" loses some of its power. Most of the time, anyway.

We have to admit, though, that once in a while we all encounter days when the MonSter presents itself so close to our faces that we can't see past its very existence. It's one big thing, too rock-solid to be broken down into manageable little pieces.

October 20 was one of those days for several of us, including Lori. At least we were able to talk about it with her and with one another.

▲▲▲

DEE — Lori, I know exactly what you mean about wanting some control back in your life. But how to get it? I guess we can't really control anything in our lives as far as disease, death, some say taxes, our grown children, and sometimes our little children, etc.

We are very vulnerable as people, as human beings. I guess we just learn how to cope as we go along.

But, Lori, don't feel bad for getting your feelings out. How many times have you all told me that? March must have been a bad month, because that is when most of my trouble started, too.

It must be very difficult, having this and being only twenty-eight. I can't imagine. I'm fifty-four and I hate it. There are so many things I can't do now that I used to do with ease. Sometimes I just don't get it.

▲▲▲

LORI — Dee, I think you just nailed it. We're vulnerable. That is a very scary word and not one that I, after having to act and be strong for so many years, even like to pretend exists. I guess I can't go forward until I admit I am vulnerable and not indestructible. Nothing has ever really gotten in my way before. I have never had to admit that I might be weak. I have always been strong, and fought tooth and nail to stay that way. I have always overcome and controlled and/or manipulated things to make sure I did.

At least I know what I have to do. I have to stop fighting it and adjust. God, that just sounds so weak and like I'm giving in. It feels like I am quitting. Do you ever get over that feeling of defeat?

▲▲▲

JOY — Maybe not entirely, Lori, but it does get easier to deal with. Yesterday I tried to lead an almost-normal day: up at 8:30 A.M., despite not getting to sleep until almost 3 A.M., and then swept the patio, did three loads of laundry, and spent some time on the phone talking about new houses. *No nap!* By 6 P.M., I barely had the strength to feed the dogs their dinner. Took my meds, talked to Jack at length about whether we should make an offer on the new house we've been looking at, and fell into bed around midnight.

But this morning, I got up early, briefly, just to tend to the dogs, and then crawled back into bed and didn't get up until noon. Even then, I wanted to stay where I was, and I had to force myself to get up. So I'm half a day behind already with things I wanted to do. But I had to face the fact that my body is protesting the treatment it got yesterday, and I *must* take it easier today. It sucks.

At some point, we have to re-prioritize and give "Listening to Body" the highest priority. Body, mind, and spirit have to work in harmony, work together, or everything gets even more out of whack. Often, in our cases, "the spirit is willing, but the flesh is weak." So we have to compromise. Today I feel a bit frustrated, but not defeated. As Scarlett said, "Tomorrow is another day!"

▲▲▲

DEE — Lori, I believe there is a difference between defeat and acceptance. Acceptance is strength and defeat is not. A man in our apartment building recently died of Lou Gehrig's (ALS) disease. He was not really old, just sixty-seven. When he first moved here, about a year ago, he knew he had something wrong, but he had no diagnosis yet. In a few weeks, he found out he had ALS and had six to nine months to live.

He accepted this, was depressed about it sometimes, and reacted in a human way, but he got his affairs in order, got his spirit ready, got his family together. Basically, he faced his illness with a bravery that I doubt I will ever reach. He was an inspiration to us all.

I'm certainly not saying that you shouldn't vent. That is one of the reasons for our Froup. I know I need it. Mostly, I related this to show what I meant by acceptance rather than defeat.

▲▲▲

ME — Lori, adjusting to something, anything, but especially something that hits at your essential being, is not a weakness. The time comes when you have to adjust to it, unless you have a particular fondness for beating your head against a wall. This has more to do with accepting and adapting than with "giving in." It takes a lot of courage and creativity to find ways of continuing to be a viable, vital wife, mother, employee, whatever, when there are so many obstacles thrown in front of you. You have a right to feel tired, frustrated, depressed—that's where you find the motivation to develop new ways of "doing." It's okay for you to be down right now. We know for sure that you'll be back to your old whipping and snapping soon. And that's all that's required of you, that you just keep on being you, with whatever changes you have to make to make life easier.

▲▲▲

RENEE — Lori, I hate feeling vulnerable. I would rather run naked in the street, on live television, eating big, long, runny worms, than feel vulnerable. Something about me just keeps trying to present myself as Superwoman. I've gotten better, but I have such a long, long way to go in this department. Vulnerable is still how I feel when I have to ask someone to help me.

I know a couple of things, Lori—you have not given up and you will not give up. It ain't in you to do that, honey, so you can forget it. And though you believe you have given up, that doesn't make it a fact. It's just a feeling—did I get that right, Sharon? [Sharon, our Froup therapist, is usually the one to point out when a reaction is "just a feeling."] And yes, you can get control back into your life. The only thing is, it's a different life. And guess what, it can actually be better than the old one!

▲▲▲

KIM — Today is one of those days I *hate* having MS. Nothing in my freaking body is working right. I had the most horrific spasms in my right leg at lunchtime today. Since then my whole right side has been fucked up. I almost fell on my face about six times.

I don't like it. I don't like it! I *hate* it! It sucks. I sure wish it would just go away. Please, someone. . . . Damn, and now I can't even type. When I ain't peeing or shitting my pants, I am tripping on my own feet. I guess I am lucky that what is happening this time is on my right side, since I am a leftie! So what next? I guess call the neurologist on Monday, but she will say the same old shit again. "Let's do I.V.s" or something. I just want the whole thing to go away and let us get back to our old lives.

Have you guys ever had a flare-up and felt, or just kind of knew, that things weren't going to get a lot better? Like a premonition. I had a feeling years before I even had symptoms that I was going to get MS. Now I have the feeling that things aren't going to get a whole lot easier or better. I'm not complaining (not right this second). I'm just feeling a little frustrated and a lot afraid. How do you all do it? Cope, I mean, plan, whatever it takes not to fall apart. Make career decisions, etc!?

▲▲▲

ME AGAIN — I've been trying for forever to figure this one out. I guess each of us has to assess our own health situations, resources, abilities, and whatever we need to enable us to identify our goals and move toward them. We might even have to rethink our goals. I think the best thing is to just do it a day at a time, or a minute at a time, or whatever it takes. I know that sounds like buying into a cliché, but the truth of it hits home once in a while.

I find that if I go beyond the immediate future with my plans, I set myself up for disappointment and frustration. I find it helpful, when I have to make plans for something, to have a plan A and a plan B as backup. Usually, there's a way of having both work out in the end. Like when I decided to go back to writing. Or trying to write. I kind of told myself, if I'm not able to write a book, I'll at least read ten books. I'm nearly finished with both now. It has taken an almost supreme effort (and the help of twenty-some kindred souls). But it's a way to keep on keeping on, even when there's a lot of failure involved (and there has been!). Experiencing failures is worthwhile if it gives me a chance to face them and remake them into something constructive.

I know I'm spouting a bunch of platitudes here. I guess you all are challenging me to face and remake my problems in the light of your own searches for ways to cope. Hang in there! (That's another platitude, but what else can we do?)

▲▲▲

RENEE — Yep, Kimmers, I know all about the game of "just knowing" that things aren't gonna get a lot better. After reading your letter, I sat for a few minutes and verbalized to myself (actually said it out loud) that, without divine intervention of some sort, I will never again be without symptoms of multiple sclerosis. Somewhere, awhile back, I crossed the line between having periods of no symptoms and then flare-ups into always having symptoms that are getting worse and then having flare-ups on top of that. I guess this is what is meant by the term "secondary progressive"—who knows? I don't say all this in a complaining way, either; I am just stating what I believe is now true for me. Strangely enough, when I said it out loud, I didn't start crying, get depressed, or feel kicked in the gut.

Actually, when I was feeling so bad a couple of weeks ago, I discovered something that helps. I was reading some of the mail from y'all, not just the letters saying y'all are hoping that I get better, but the letters about how y'all are doing. Reading the letters about *you* and not about *me* is what makes me feel better. And I just realized that I feel better when I worry about somebody besides myself. That was a very uplifting discovery. Which makes me believe even more firmly that there is a purpose for all of us being alive—just look what y'all did for me. Thank you from the bottom of my heart.

I'm now going back to reading mail and thinking good thoughts.

▲▲▲

TARA — When I was in my twenties, I "knew" that I was going to have problems that would be visible at some point. I think that part of that knowledge came from feeling so darn lousy all the time. I mean, I just knew that no one could feel as bad as I did and not expect it to show at some point. When my ex-hubby and I built our house, I insisted on bigger bathrooms and wider doorways and all that stuff so that it would remain accessible to me for life. I'm sure that he thought I was a hypochondriac, but I *knew* that I was going to get worse. I honestly think that he knew, too, but he didn't want to believe it.

Kim and Lynn and all, I can relate to the question about how we plan and carry on, etc., etc. Hmm, that's a good question, and one that has given me my moments, that's for sure. You know, all my life I thought, gee, I am going to make this huge difference in the world. Yet I was not sure if all that I did was really that beneficial to everybody involved.

Then, a couple of years ago, I made it my long-term plan to demonstrate joy in all that I do, in anything that is handed to me, through all of it. Now that I just try to bring others love and joy, well, I can see the effects that it has on others. So I dumped the long-term plans, the "I am going to save the world" creed. Now I just go with joy wherever I find myself.

I have to admit that there are times when I think, *okay!* Enough already! Mostly, though, I just live in the present and take whatever comes my way as part of the ride. I know that I can't control my life, because as soon as I try, the old MS comes up and changes everything around me. So I just automatically think, hmmm, I guess this is happening because I wasn't supposed to do that, or go in that direction, or whatever. So I go in the new direction and take a close look at where it is leading me, and it is always okay.

Now, I guess I don't have to tell any of you that I don't sit passively, either. But I don't beat my head against the wall over and over like I used to. If I know that something is going to wear me down and is just too much for me, I say so. Then I let it go, no matter what others think.

One time my mom and I researched all the resources that were in the area for people with MS-type conditions. We looked at the worst-case scenario and called around and found out everything that is out there that I might be able to access someday. By doing that, I developed a plan that I can fall back on if I need this or that kind of help in my life. And Plan B is the "go live with Mom and Dad" choice. I know that it is there if I need it.

I guess all I am saying is that I know that there will be hard times, and there will be times that for the life of us we can't figure out why the heck we're going through this. At those times, it is okay to scream and say, "I hate this MS!"

Other than that, I don't try to plan my future too far in advance. I do think of possibilities that I might go toward, but I don't dwell on it too much beyond that.

▲▲▲

BARB —Kim, just take it one baby step at a time!

I don't make decisions anymore. I just ride the tide until the outcome hits me in the face. I used to be such a complete control freak; I drove everyone crazy, including myself. Now I have learned, to some extent, to go with the flow. I sometimes think that's part of the lesson I am to learn from all of this. I don't believe that we are afflicted because of anything any of us did—don't get me wrong. But I do think there are lessons to be learned in every phase we go through and everything we experience in this life.

It can be very tempting to make a quick decision so that you can get on with what you have to do, or to be done with something and feel some closure. But, Kim, take some time, don't be too hasty. Things have been kind of troublesome and crashing down on you lately (on many of us, actually), so try to slide for just a bit and see if you feel the same in a few days or weeks or even months. This MonSter is nothing if not changeable and unpredictable!

▲▲▲

VICKI — Man, talk about some heavy-duty reading today! It looks like several of us had to vent. We should all be a lot healthier for it!

I went with Larry to pick up Ashley after the game last night. I sat in the truck while he went to the field to get her. As I sat watching some of the other parents leave with their kids, I noticed how easy it was for them to walk. Just walk. No speed walking, no skipping. Just walking with ease. A second-nature type of thing. It felt so odd to watch them. It was almost funny to see these people and the simplest things that we all take/ took for granted.

I made the comment once that I wished I had twins. Well, I got them. I read an article on MS before I was diagnosed, and I thought to myself, if I have to have something later on, at least MS isn't fatal. I wouldn't mind having something like that. Well, I got it.

Sometimes I'm afraid of feeling too good. If I just feel okay, I don't get knocked so far down when another flare-up hits. If I feel great, I hit bottom really hard when the flare-ups come. The reality of it hits me like a huge slap in the face.

In some ways, I am thankful that I have MS. It has slowed me down a lot. I now notice things like grasses in the ditch that others call weeds. I feed the doves that others hunt. I truly think I now "see" things that others may not. I am a nicer person than I used to be.

I wonder what I'd do if somebody found a 'cure.' I wonder if I'll go back to my old self if I'm cured. That scares the hell out of me.

Lori, Kim, everybody, make the best damn lemonade you can out of those lemons that have been thrown into your lap. Remember, on our headstones, the only thing that matters is the dash between the dates!

▲▲▲

DONNA — When I try to deal with MS, every time I reach a level of acceptance, something new crops up or something old decides to intensify. I strive to be good and live by all the old platitudes, but sometimes I just have to vent. Sometimes I have to push against the disease. Sometimes I have to hate it enough to keep fighting. Sometimes I can say, "Okay, I've got it. So what?" But every time that I can recall that I have said, "I can deal with this," I'm knocked to my knees with an exacerbation.

Writing used to be my salvation. My writing has helped me through many crises and has helped me understand who I am. For some reason, though, it has been very difficult for me to write in my journal about this disease. I can write to the Froup, to each of you individually or as a whole. I can talk about it with anyone I choose. But I cannot sit down and write about the disease for myself. I've started to write almost every day, but I've marked through more than I've left undisturbed. I am puzzled by this, but I know that when the time is right, I will write until I run out of words.

I know that this too shall pass. . . . I'm just not too sure about that meatloaf I had for dinner last night!

▲▲▲

SHARON — I felt depressed and afraid when I was told, "Hey, fool, you've got MS!" And the last few years before that statement were rough by anyone's standards. But I think that "rough" is a relative term, as is "normal." MS won't interfere with our lives all that much as long as we pay attention, stay emotionally available to ourselves (most of all) and our families and friends, and make the necessary adjustments. Sometimes we might not get a choice on that; but what the hell, that's life with or without multiple sclerosis. And yes, we'll have days, like today, when we will grieve, even though we would all rather eat dirt. But grieving can feel good sometimes, y'know?

Hang in there, everybody. One thing MS can never do is rob us of our love of life.

▲▲▲

RENEE — Lori, everybody else that's having a rough day—I've had that feeling that I am weak and giving in. Like I am a quitter. I think I got rid of that feeling about the time I decided that maybe I ought to start thinking that life and everything in it is a challenge. And since I have never been one to turn down a challenge or a bet, I found myself getting a little excited about ways to adjust. Since I wanted to be MS poster girl of the month, I figured I'd better come up with some really great ideas on how to live with MS. It sure kept me busy, and still does. I didn't make poster girl. But that doesn't matter, because my thinking started to change, a little slowly at first, but then it kind of picked up speed when I really let myself go.

So yes, you will get over the feeling of defeat, and I know you will rise to the challenge. And you will most likely teach all of us a few things that will help us, because you are all ladies who love adventure. When you start looking forward to the challenges, even if that means just being able to make it to the mailbox, you will get stronger. You'll have some bad days, sure, but you *will* also have good ones. And whether you know it or not, you already have the control over your life that you so desperately are seeking. We all have some control over our lives. If we didn't, we would not be able to write all that we've shared with one another. We would just sit. And do absolutely nothing.

Okay, I am getting off my soapbox or whatever they call that thing (not podium, please). Just know that we all are right here with you and you are gonna do better than you can even believe. When the bad days hit, we can't seem to remember the good ones, and then we think they might never come back again. They will. Pretty soon bad days won't be so bad, because you will really believe another good one is around the corner. Trust me. It happens all the time.

18

Parting Thoughts

The members of our Froup responded to my requests for input or gave me permission to use information I'd already received from them, on each of the tiny aspects of going through life hand-in-hand with the MonSter. After collecting all these anecdotal tidbits, I was curious to know what some of our ladies considered most important to tell others about this journey as a whole. So I asked the Flutterbuds what final thought they'd each like to leave with anybody looking for information on life with multiple sclerosis or other chronic disorders, what general "overview" they'd like readers to carry away with them, or perhaps what bit of advice they'd like to give to those newly diagnosed and just beginning to meet the challenges that we've all faced for various numbers of years. Here are some of their (and my) responses:

▲▲▲

SHARON — As MS started to take its toll on my body, I began to pass through several stages of grief and loss—pain has a tendency to drive one closer to her Higher Power, open her up to introspection. As a result, I was forced to slow down. I have asked for direction and followed the path. I now take the time to look for another open door instead of beating my head, until I bleed and my soul is wounded, against the one that has just closed. I'm not exactly sure yet why I was given the gift of MS. There are times when I think that it gives me a better understanding of others' weaknesses and frailties. It has given me the gift of relaxation; it's amazing that I couldn't relax until I had to!

Since I have slowed down, I can take the time to listen to the still, small voice inside me and to really feel my connection to the planet instead of just understanding the concept.

▲▲▲

DEE — I have also learned that it is good to slow down and enjoy what each day brings. Some days it's difficult, due to pain or new symptoms or frustration over the inability to do some of things I want to do. But enjoying a new grandchild or some flowers or animals or family or friends takes time and some effort. Frankly, I think that is what this world needs—for us to stop and think about what this great gift of life is all about and to be thankful for being a part of it, in whatever way we're still able.

I think all illness, especially chronic illness, causes a deep sense of loss. It's normal, I think, to remember how things used to be or how they would/could have been, to long for the days when we weren't affected by disease. But I believe this loss would happen anyway, even without MS. It happens with aging, when we can't do the things we once did, when we lose someone we love. Loss is a part of living. There are definite gains in dealing with all of this: a deep sense of appreciation for all that we do have and a great amount of compassion for others who suffer. Some people never have the opportunity to learn that. Now that's a big loss, even though they may not realize it.

▲▲▲

KIM — I have thought and thought and thought about how MS has changed my life. Usually, my answer would depend on the day or the week that you asked that question. Sometimes I would feel bitter. Why did this have to happen to me? Then again, why not? I guess if I have to sum up how it has changed me, this is my answer:

First, it has made me a far more honest person. I tell people what I am going through. It took me six years to figure out how to do this. Now I am pretty honest about it, maybe even to a fault. I want people to understand. I want them to learn about it. It has, I hope, made me more passionate and compassionate in my work. I try to understand more of what my patients are going through and what their families are feeling. I try to understand their side of things instead of thinking they are just bitchy families!

It has made me appreciate the small things all the more. I used to thrive on *big* paychecks. Now I understand that with a big paycheck comes less energy to spend it (although I admit that more money and less work would be a *great* alternative!). I love sunny days! I love taking a ride and not spending the whole day running around. I love the days that Dad and I go out and buy each other milkshakes and onion rings at our favorite little dive. Mostly, I love the thought that maybe I'm making my mother proud by dealing with this all in the best way that I know how. [N.B.: Kim's mother died the day after Kim was diagnosed with MS.] I hope that she is proud of me! And I love all the people that I have gotten to know in this group. Without MS, that wouldn't have happened!

▲▲▲

I guess the most important thing I'd like to pass on, especially to others who are new to life with the MonSter, is that nothing about MS is carved in stone. Days of struggle and depression can be followed by as many days of triumph and exhilaration. A treatment that worked for years may all of a sudden become ineffective. On the other hand, a medication that did zilch on a first or second try might suddenly work miracles.

I've learned to refrain from making predictions about how far the disease will progress in me, how quickly that will happen, or what effects it will have on my life in general. So far, my condition is both much worse than I'd hoped and much better than I'd expected. As soon as I make any proclamations about my status quo, it changes. If I brag about how well I'm doing, I soon end up having to push myself through a sudden fog, bound by fatigue, numbness, pain, and depression. If I bemoan my condition, I turn around and find myself able to keep turning around, when five minutes before I'd been close to paralysis. If I allow myself a moment of weakness when I curse God for "letting" this happen to me, I see a sign of his power at work in and through my difficulties.

I think I've learned that, even as I write a book about multiple sclerosis, making myself concentrate solely on it for a number of hours every day, MS doesn't have to be the guiding influence in my life for the rest of that day. If I concentrate mostly on the other forces in my life, multiple sclerosis falls into place as something generally manageable, almost insignificant, in the hierarchy of my priorities.

▲▲▲

SHARON — I used to wonder if I would get sicker if I focused on the negative aspects of my disease (I don't even care to refer to it as that; it's just a "temporarily-out-of-order" issue for me). I'm not what I consider "all that bad." I'm still walking, exercising, able to deal with running a home, etc., etc. But as time goes on, I am able to see that I do have an illness, and that I'd better pay attention to it or it will sneak up behind me and bite me in the ass.

I've thought about what I would do if a cure for MS came along (didn't we get into a discussion on this another time?), and I got this weird little feeling in my belly: fear. Since I've invested so much in learning to deal with this disease or "gift" from God (depending on what kind of day I'm having—sometimes I call it my "shining affliction"), I'm not so sure how I would feel. It would take a while to fill that space in me that MS has taken up for so long.

Now don't get me wrong. If there was a cure, I would be the first to go for it. Just imagine, no more worrying about blindness or the ability to walk or to go to the bathroom with dignity or getting intention tremors in both hands or continuous numbness and spasms that keep us awake at night, and, of course, the depression and fatigue.

So what *would* we fill that space with? A little relief from fear and worry? Maybe! Time spent doing the things we love but couldn't do because of fatigue? I would! Stop wondering what I will do if my eyes go or both hands quit operating and won't do a damned thing I say? Sounds good to me!

But multiple sclerosis has become a part of me, a part that has shed new light on relationships new and old, a part that has given me introspection that I don't think would have come about without MS, a part that has created a lifestyle change, from believing I was all-powerful to acknowledging that I am both empowered and vulnerable. It has brought a little honesty into my life and showed me that pride and dignity do not come from a perfect body and a fat wallet. It has taught me that I am lovable despite my frailties, and that I am perfectly imperfect; I don't think I would be who I am if MS had not entered my life and I had not paid attention to its encouragement to change.

I do know that there is more than a disease holding this Froup of lunatics together, so I don't think we have anything to worry about as far as a cure making us lose touch with one another. Just think of the celebration!

▲▲▲

JANE — I think we're talking about coming to terms with the changes MS brings. There are without a doubt many losses.

Nevertheless, *no one* and *nothing* can take the essence of who we are from us. Some people would call it the soul. Whatever name we give it, it is what distinguishes each of us from every other person in this world. It is a uniqueness, and it remains and grows despite the MS and its circumstances. It's the part of us that brought us to the edge of living, and that now can be transformed into stamina and the drive to press forward with a new style of living. We each have something vital that we can and must now channel toward productive life-giving. We must make a decision toward *life*.

Another way to see it is as a decision to carry on, to say *yes* to living and living well, despite the smacks MS or life in general bring about. God (by whatever name you choose to call him) delights in our turning to him for strength and sustenance, and he will readily provide. I think the biggest help is to realize that we are *not* alone in this, and to allow others to minister to us in all ways, just as we continue to give to others.

▲▲▲

KIM — There's something that I would like to add. I don't know how to put it, exactly. But something that has scared me to death in being part of a group like this is the sharing of bad experiences that come with MS. When I had my first big attack, I almost chose not to have the I.V. steroid treatment because of some of the experiences I'd heard about from the people here. I think that somewhere we should clarify that these *are* the worst experiences. MS does not affect all people in the same way. Nor are the side effects of different medications or treatments the same for all of us.

▲▲▲

RENEE — I was officially diagnosed with MS in December 1986. I immediately read everything about MS that I could get my hands on, which was probably one of the biggest mistakes of my life. Most of it was outdated. All of it sounded like a bunch of gloom and doom. There was a lot about bad experiences with bad treatments.

Fortunately, doctors and researchers know more about MS now. The outlook in terms of progression through the stages of MS has taken a radical turn for the better. It is true that my health is worse than it was since my diagnosis; in fact, it is worse than it was even a year ago. However, I am still mobile, I am still capable of taking care of myself as well as my ten-year-old grandson, whom I have raised since birth. Some days are great, some days are not so great, but there are *no* days that I can't handle, because I have God in my life. No, I am not religious (although I certainly have nothing against religion); I am what I call "spiritual."

There have been numerous accounts for quite some time of people who have chosen assisted suicide. Whether this is morally or legally wrong is not my concern. But I am very opposed to the way that the media has continued to report that so many of the people who chose suicide had been diagnosed with MS. It seems they could simply say the person was ill and leave it at that.

I want to scream from the highest rooftop, *"Please* do not assume that MS is going to kill you, make you bedridden, take away your ability to speak or walk or otherwise function. Please do not believe everything you read. While there are certainly lots of people that seem to have the all the symptoms from time to time, remember that you may not ever lose your ability to walk (for example) simply because someone else with MS has lost that ability. Even if you do, you could very easily wake up one morning and be able to walk again. Symptoms can come and go. Very few of them ever stay forever (read the statistics). And if you do find that someday you are somewhat more limited than you were before, you can and will adjust."

I truly believe that at some point in the near future there will be a cure for MS. Medical experts are working around the clock in an effort to achieve that goal. They have already made great strides in developing medications that can slow down the disease in a large number of people.

As hard as it may seem at first, please try to get involved in a support group of people who have MS [see the Resources section at the end of the book]. They know first-hand everything that you're going through. They can offer you experience, strength, and hope in ways that *only* a person with MS can. It was hard for me to even go to a support group meeting in the beginning, because I saw people who used canes or wheelchairs. Somehow I missed the other 90 percent of the people in the room who truly "looked so good."

The group I'm with now (online) has more than twenty other women who all have MS. I have never in all my life found a group of people (any kind of group, MS or otherwise) who are as close and intertwined in every aspect of one another's lives as we are. Surprisingly, most of us have never seen one another in real life. But we laugh together, cry together, share all our fears and triumphs, and, above all else, love each other unconditionally. I cannot imagine going through life (even if I did not have MS) without the strength and support that I continue to receive from these very special people.

So, please don't give up just because you've been diagnosed with MS. No matter who you are, there is always going to be someone who comes into your life who can give you the strength, the benefit of their experience, and the hope that you need. And there will be those that need the strength, experience, and hope that only you can give them. You may be the thread they hold onto when everything else seems to have failed them. If you are not there for them, if you do not reach out and just share a smile, I believe that all of us in this world would suffer in the long run. We'd lose out on the miracle of two human beings who are able to truly connect and share on a level that most people never experience in their entire lives. I think this is the way God intended us to reach out to one another.

▲▲▲

I want to believe, as Renee does, that a cure for MS is on the horizon, and that I'll welcome it when it happens. But I have to agree with Sharon, too, that the idea of a cure can be scary. As is true of so many others in the Froup, I've gotten used to having the Monster as my constant (more constant now than ever before) companion. Sometimes I think that I'm going through what many kidnap victims report: as time goes on, the initial horror of their bondage becomes blunted, to the point that the captivity itself seems to be a kind of sanctuary. I, too, wonder what would take over my life if the MS someday disappeared. It's so hard for me to admit that I even have these thoughts. For example, I often say that I'm jealous of people who are able to work outside their homes. Yet, after all this time, I know I'd be terrified to get behind the wheel of a car, drive to an office, and face the daily routine and the constant challenge of employment. I guess that I've been forced to make my present life a safe place to be, and any hint of change is frightening.

I also tend to defend myself against letting hope for a cure invade my self-induced complacency. I tell myself that it's never going to happen. I know that MS is an expensive disease to treat. Expensive treatments mean big money for drug companies; there's that cynical part of me that expects researchers to forever concentrate on developing more and more expensive treatments rather than looking for a cure. Yet even as I try to muster up a respectable measure of anger at the drug manufacturers, there's another part of me that truly believes in the honest, committed, benevolent scientists at work right now. Their efforts will, without a doubt, result in the magic formula for a cure very soon.

▲▲▲

PAT — I remember a time when the MonSter was on the attack in me, trying to take away everything that I held dear. At least at the time, I thought it was the MonSter that was doing it. But, after a year of struggling and pushing and struggling some more, I found that this MonSter can't take away anything that I won't let it take from me.

Six months after my diagnosis, I was in a wheelchair and was not expected to ever walk again. I was put on I.V. steroids, medications galore, the whole bit. I gained weight, looked fat, and felt ugly and generally unacceptable as a human being. I spent hours writing letters to my husband and children, apologizing for being so useless to them. In other words, I was a MeSs.

Then, one day while I was sitting around doing nothing, feeling as low as low can get, I started to get mad. Mad at this thing that was taking away my life. Mad at the doctors who give such grim diagnoses.

I decided then that no way in hell was this beast going to take away any more of my life! I struggled to walk, and I fell. I struggled some more, and I fell. I continued to struggle for about a year, and one day the struggle turned into a small triumph. Each day got a little easier. Soon I was wheelchair-free! That was almost eighteen years ago. I still use my crutches, my handicapped placard, the standard "accessories." But not the wheelchair.

And I've stopped writing letters of apology to my family. I've ripped up those old ones from years ago. When I read them over, I realized that it was fear talking, not the real "me." Some of them were darned depressing, I have to admit. Still, I'm glad I was able to express my fear and let it all out. That's the first step in saying, "The hell with this MonSter! I've got a life and I'm going to live it!" It may take some doing, but the rest will come. We get through what we need to get through to get on with living. There are good days ahead!

▲▲▲

Pat has, I think, touched on something that is essential in living with MS and similar chronic, progressive disorders. Although it might seem that all control of our lives has been wrenched from us, we are still allowed to choose to accept and to make the most of the good that lies ahead. We are still blessed with reason to hope that the good days Pat talks about are waiting for each of us.

Thank God that most of us, most of the time, are able to hold onto that bit of hope! I think we were and are blessed that we've had one another to buoy that hope.

▲▲▲

DONNA — Each of you is testimony that life can be lived despite the MonSter. I don't know where I'd be or how I'd feel about this disease if I hadn't been able to communicate with all of you about it. Even if I didn't always LOL or ROFL [laugh out loud or roll on the floor laughing], I still found a reason to smile and sometimes even chuckle.

▲▲▲

JANIS — For me, the best way to cope is to remember that when one door is closed, a new one is opened. Don't ever be afraid to step through that new opening and continue in life. Make the best of life with what you have, and experience it all to the fullest. Always look ahead to a better way and a better place. Take it one day at a time, minute by minute, whatever it takes.

▲▲▲

JAMIE — Back at the beginning, after my diagnosis, if I had just accepted that I would get worse and would have to stop everything because I have MS and don't want to be "stared at" and don't want people to notice that I have a disability, I might as well have died!

Maybe I'm just crazy, but I have had more fun, laughter, love, tears, compassion, and overall life-fulfilling events since MS than before. Life is made up of a mosaic of the good, the bad, and the indifferent day-to-day lessons. Who more than we has learned to take *nothing* for granted, to rise above trials and tribulations, and to truly feel for our fellow human beings? I think we know, really *know*, that something somewhere is so powerful that, even in our darkest moments, we are renewed with strength and with the desire to continue on the journey. We choose to help others along the way, too, with a smile, a hug, a kiss, a listening ear, or just a simple prayer that says, "Thank you, God, for giving me today."

▲▲▲

JANE

Gifted

The soft kiss of a balmy spring breeze
. . . Cotton wafts of heaven
. . . Fluffed just right
. . . I still have that to enjoy.
Graceful, delicate bends of the dogwood
. . . Pastel pink, picture-perfect
. . . Dotted bits of lace
. . . Greet me when I turn.
Children swinging in the schoolyard
. . . Brilliant colors scurry
. . . So much forgotten energy
. . . Those carefree, golden days.
I watch, I love, I feel, I hope, I am.
There's a lot of living left to do.

Resources

Organizations

National Multiple Sclerosis Society
1-800-FIGHTMS

This is the national office in New York. They provide information, educational materials, and referrals to other helpful sources.

The national office can also provide location information and phone numbers for branch chapters throughout the United States. Contact your closest chapter for information about self-help and support groups, rental or loan of durable medical equipment, physical therapy, respite care, peer counseling, family counseling, and many other services. The society also has volunteer opportunities for MS patients and anybody else who is interested.

Books

David L. Carroll and Jon Dudley Dorman, M.D., *Living Well With MS: A Guide for Patient, Caregiver and Family* (New York: HarperCollins, 1993).

Marion Deutsche Cohen and Mary Wyngaarden Krauss, *Dirty Details: The Days and Nights of a Well Spouse* (Philadelphia, PA: Temple University Press, 1996).

Nancy J. Holland, T. Jock Murray and Stephen C. Reingold, *Multiple Sclerosis: A Guide for the Newly Diagnosed* (New York: Demos Vermande, 1996).

Rosalind C. Kalb, Ph.D., *Multiple Sclerosis: The Questions You Have, The Answers You Need* (New York: Demos Vermande, 1996).

Richard Lechtenberg, M.D., *Multiple Sclerosis Fact Book* (Philadelphia, PA: F. A. Davis Company, 1995).

Louis J. Rosner and Shelley Ross, *Multiple Sclerosis: New Hope and Practical Advice for People with MS and Their Families* (New York: Simon & Schuster, 1992).

Phillip D. Rumrill, Jr., *Employment Issues and Multiple Sclerosis* (New York: Demos Vermande, 1996).

Barbara D. Webster, *All of a Piece: A Life with Multiple Sclerosis* (Baltimore, MD: Johns Hopkins University Press, 1990).

Many other suggestions are at:
http://members.aol.com/healthbooks/ms/

Internet Resources

MSers with Internet access have almost limitless stores of information available to them. Entering the words "multiple sclerosis" in a search will produce more links to MS material than can be viewed at one (or two or three or . . . sittings). Here are the addresses of a few **websites** on which to begin browsing:

National Multiple Sclerosis Society
www.nmss.org

Med Support FSF International
www.healthboards.com

The International MS Support Foundation
www.msnews.org/

Johns Hopkins Intelihealth News
www.intelihealth.com

Thrive!
www.Thriveonline.com

Each of these sites is connected with still other sites by hyperlinks. You can click on any of them to access more facts about MS.

The **Internet message boards** are a good place to talk with other MSers. It seems that there is a site on every Internet server where MSers can share information, ask questions, get answers, let off steam, and make friends.

I've only used **America Online**—if that's your server, go to the MS area by typing in the keywords "better health" and then follow the prompts to the message boards. This site also gives information on scheduled chat groups.

Compuserve's MS information center and bulletin boards are at http://go.compuserve.com/multiplesclerosis.

For **other servers**, using "multiple sclerosis" as the keywords and then following the prompts will probably eventually take you to wherever you want to go.

The **International MS Support Foundation** (http://www. msnews.org) is an independent, non-profit organization founded to improve the understanding of MS through education, and to reduce isolation by providing a support network for patients, their families, friends, and physicians. The IMSSF publishes newsletters and offers other services, including sponsoring message boards for people with MS and their caregivers at http://aspin.asu.edu/msnews/bb.

Forming an Internet Group

The boards are also the best place to go if you are interested in forming a group like the Flutterbuds. The ladies in our Froup all started out just reading and answering on the message boards. After several months, we kind of gravitated to one another, with no real plans for that to happen. We (Renee was the first to say it cyber-aloud) realized at a certain point that we each needed to talk with certain ladies on the boards much more than others. I think that this was happening naturally already, so that people who visited the boards less frequently and weren't able to keep track of a lot of one-on-one or -two or-three conversations began to feel left out (it's true; they were!). It was clear that everybody would be more comfortable if we quietly moved off by ourselves. (We still go back to the boards occasionally to talk with the other people we met there.)

Forming a Froup (or whatever you'll call it) can't be forced, of course. It works the same way as forming a "real" group of like-minded members. It will happen when it's supposed to, if it's supposed to. It might only take a suggestion, like Renee's, that interested parties meet in a chat room (which can be set up for this purpose) at a certain time on a certain day. It's likely that the people who show up will be the very ones that you, or the "Renee" on your board, wanted to "go independent" with.

If a Froup doesn't "happen," that's okay, too. The message boards are still great places to share support, advice, encouragement, and, ultimately, real friendship with the people who really understand: other MSers!

Glossary

ACTH: adrenocorticotrophic hormone, a medication administered to MSers, usually by intravenous infusions or intramuscular injections, to stimulate the body to produce cortisone, thereby reducing acute inflammation in the central nervous system

Amantadine: unclassified therapeutic agent, used in management of multiple sclerosis to relieve fatigue and prevent certain viral illnesses

baclofen: muscle relaxant used to reduce spasticity in multiple sclerosis and other spinal cord disorders

benign/sensory MS: a form of MS that affects/impairs sense of touch, with little or no loss of function

celiac disease: chronic nutritional disturbance caused by poor absorption of nutrients; results in diarrhea, malnutrition, and/or distended abdomen

Cylert: a central nervous system stimulant

evoked potential tests: used to measure the speed of the brain's response to visual, auditory, and sensory stimuli

exacerbations: periodic attacks during which new multiple sclerosis symptoms appear, old ones reappear, or existing ones get worse

fibromyalgia: painful disorder affecting widespread areas of the musculoskeletal system; frequently diagnosed in MSers

intention tremor: spastic movement induced by conscious effort to use the hands to perform a particular task

lesions: spotty areas on brain and spinal cord in which myelin has been destroyed, visible by MRI (see below)

Lhermitte's sign: electric shock like sensation running from the back of the head down the spine and into the extremities, brought on by flexing the neck or other sudden movements; present in many disorders involving the spinal cord

lupus: systemic lupus erythematosis; autoimmune disease involving joint pain, sun sensitivity, and/or central nervous system symptoms; early signs may be confused with those of MS

MRI: magnetic resonance imaging, a test that provides an anatomical picture of the brain and spinal cord; used to locate lesions caused by myelin loss in multiple sclerosis

myasthenia gravis: chronic illness characterized by abnormal muscle weakness and fatigue

myelin: fatty covering on nervous system; destruction of myelin interrupts pathways from brain to nerves, producing symptoms of multiple sclerosis

neurogenic bladder: disorder characterized by bladder spasms, retention of urine, incontinence; neurological in origin

NSAID: nonsteroidal anti-inflammatory drug, used to relieve pain and inflammation; available by prescription and in over-the-counter formulations (ibuprofen, naproxyn)

optic neuritis (ON): inflammation of the optic nerve, characterized by severe pain and various visual disturbances; common early symptom of multiple sclerosis

oxybutynin: prescription medication used to relieve bladder spasticity, especially in spinal cord disorders such as multiple sclerosis

plaque: sclerotic areas (covered with scar tissue) on brain and spinal cord; presence (seen on MRI) in more than one area is evidence of multiple sclerosis

prednisone: steroid drug widely used to reduce central nervous system inflammation during exacerbations of MS; in various forms, it can be administered orally, by intramuscular injection, or, most commonly, by a three- to five-day series of intravenous infusions

Prozac: prescription antidepressant

remitting/relapsing (or relapsing/remitting) stage: stage of multiple sclerosis characterized by periods of new or worsening symptoms followed by periods during which symptoms improve or disappear

rightsided (or leftsided) spasticity: jerky, uncontrollable movement on one side of the body

Ritalin: central nervous system stimulant

serotonin: organic compound found in animal and human tissue, especially the brain; one of its functions is to elevate mood

spinal tap: also known as lumbar puncture; procedure in which cerebrospinal fluid is withdrawn and analyzed for presence of high levels of white blood cells, myelin basic protein, and certain antibodies, any of which may indicate multiple sclerosis

systemic lupus erythematosis: see **lupus**

trigeminal neuralgia: inflammation of facial nerves, characterized by severe pain, usually on one side of the face at a time; common symptom of multiple sclerosis

UTI: urinary tract infection

vestibular disorder: malfunction of nerves that conduct auditory stimuli to the brain; causes problems with equilibrium

Index

Hunter House
RELATED BOOKS & RESOURCES pg. 1

LIVING *BEYOND* MULTIPLE SCLEROSIS — A WOMEN'S GUIDE *by* Judith Lynn Nichols and her Online Group of MS Sisters. Foreword by Lily Jung, M.D.

They're back! The Flutterbuds — the women whose frank, funny Internet chats became the basis for *Women Living with Multiple Sclerosis* — return with a sequel that focuses on transcending the effects of MS.

Topics include sustaining positive doctor/patient relationships, latest treatments for MS, tips for choosing and using assistive devices, and preparing applications for Social Security Disability. Time, energy, and sanity saving techniques abound, and the women share pet peeves as well as new talents and interests. The book concludes with moving comments about finding ways to nourish spirit, psyche, and imagination for life beyond MS.

288 pages ... Paperback $14.95 ... Available September 2000

GET FIT WHILE YOU SIT: Easy Workouts from Your Chair *by* Charlene Torkelson

Here is a total body workout that can be done right from your chair, anywhere. It is perfect for office workers, travelers, and those with age-related movement limitations or special conditions. The book offers three programs. The *One-Hour Chair Program* is a full-body, low-impact workout that includes light aerobics and exercises to be done with or without weights. The *5-Day Short Program* features five compact workouts for those short on time. Finally, the *Ten-Minute Miracles* are a group of easy-to-do exercises perfect for anyone on the go.

160 pages ... 212 b/w photos ... Paperback $12.95 ... Hard Cover $22.95

COMPUTER AND WEB RESOURCES FOR PEOPLE WITH DISABILITIES *by* the Alliance for Technology Access

This book shows how people can use computer technology to enhance their lives. *Part One* describes conventional and assistive technologies, and gives strategies for accessing Internet resources. *Part Two* features charts organized by access needs and referenced to software, hardware, and communication aids. *Part Three* is a gold mine of Web resources, publications, support organizations, government programs, and technology vendors.

384 pages ... 40 b/w photos ... 8 charts ... Third revised edition Paperback $20.95 ... Spiral bound $27.95 ... ASCII disk $27.95

To order or for our FREE catalog call (800) 266-5592

MENOPAUSE WITHOUT MEDICINE
by Linda Ojeda, Ph.D. ... *New Fourth Edition*

Linda Ojeda broke new ground 15 years ago with this bestselling resource on menopause, giving women a clear understanding of menopausal changes and guidelines for effective self-care.

In this new edition she re-examines the hormone therapy debate; suggests natural remedies for depression, hot flashes, sexual changes, and skin and hair problems; and presents an illustrated basic exercise program. She also includes up-to-date information on natural sources of estrogen, including phytoestrogens, and how diet and personality affect mood swings.

352 pages ... 32 illus. ... 62 tables
Paperback $15.95... Hard cover $25.95

HER HEALTHY HEART: A Woman's Guide to Preventing and Reversing Heart Disease Naturally
by Linda Ojeda, Ph.D.

Heart disease is the #1 killer of American women ages 44 to 65, yet until now most of the research and attention has been given to men. This book fills this gap by addressing the unique aspects of heart disease in women and the natural ways to combat it. Dr. Ojeda explains how women can prevent heart disease whether they take hormone replacement therapy (HRT) or not. She provides detailed information on how to reduce the risk of heart disease through diet, physical activity, and stress management.

352 pages ... Paperback $14.95 ... Hard cover $24.95

MAKING LOVE BETTER THAN EVER: Reaching New Heights of Passion and Pleasure After 40
by Barbara Keesling, Ph.D.

With maturity comes the potential for a multi-faceted, soulful loving that draws from all we are to deepen our ties of intimacy and nurturing. Sex expert Barbara Keesling provides a series of exercises that demonstrate the power of touch to heighten sexual response and expand sexual potential; reduce anxiety and increase health and well-being; build self-esteem and improve body image; open the lines of communication; and promote playfulness, spontaneity, and a natural sense of joy.

208 pages ... 14 illus. ... Paperback $13.95

All prices subject to change

THE PLEASURE PRESCRIPTION: To Love, to Work, to Play — Life In the Balance by Paul Pearsall, Ph.D.

New York Times Bestseller! This bestselling book is a prescription for stressed-out lives. Dr. Pearsall maintains that contentment, wellness, and long life can be found by devoting time to family, helping others, and slowing down to savor life's pleasures. Pearsall's unique approach draws from Polynesian wisdom and his own 25 years of psychological and medical research. For readers who want to discover a way of life that promotes healthy values and living, *The Pleasure Prescription* provides the answers.

288 pages ... Paperback $13.95 ... Hard cover $23.95

Just Announced!
PARTNERS IN PLEASURE by Paul Pearsall, Ph.D.

The much-awaited sequel to *The Pleasure Prescription* is coming in March 2001 — reserve your copy now.

WRITE YOUR OWN PLEASURE PRESCRIPTION: 60 Ways to Create Balance & Joy in Your Life by Paul Pearsall, Ph.D.

Dr. Pearsall offers this companion volume to *The Pleasure Prescription* for the many readers who have written asking for ways to translate the harmony of Oceanic life to their own lives. It is full of ideas for bringing the spirit of aloha — the ability to fully connect with oneself and with others — to everyday life. He encourages readers to disengage from the headlong rush and frenzy of Western life in order to feel the pleasure that comes from a calm acceptance of the world around us and the connection we have with others.

224 pages ... Paperback ... $12.95

WRITING FROM WITHIN: A Guide to Creativity and Your Life Story Writing by Bernard Selling

Writing from Within has attracted an enthusiastic following among those wishing to write oral histories, life narratives, or autobiographies. Bernard Selling shows new and veteran writers how to free up hidden images and thoughts, employ right-brain visualization, and use language as a way to capture feelings, people, and events. The result is at once a self-help writing workbook and an exciting journey of personal discovery and creation.

320 pages ... Third Edition ... Paperback ... $17.95

ORDER FORM

10% DISCOUNT on orders of $50 or more —
20% DISCOUNT on orders of $150 or more —
30% DISCOUNT on orders of $500 or more —
On cost of books for fully prepaid orders

NAME

ADDRESS

CITY/STATE   ZIP/POSTCODE

PHONE   COUNTRY (outside of U.S.)

TITLE	QTY	PRICE	TOTAL
Women Living with Mutiple Sclerosis (paper)		@ $13.95	
Living Beyond Mutiple Sclerosis... (paper)		@ $14.95	

Prices subject to change without notice

Please list other titles below:

		@ $	
		@ $	
		@ $	
		@ $	
		@ $	
		@ $	
		@ $	

Check here to receive our book catalog ☐   FREE

Shipping Costs:
First book: $3.00 by book post ($4.50 by UPS, Priority Mail, or to ship outside the U.S.)
Each additional book: $1.00
For rush orders and bulk shipments call us at (800) 266-5592

TOTAL _____
Less discount @_____% (_____)
TOTAL COST OF BOOKS _____
Calif. residents add sales tax _____
Shipping & handling _____
TOTAL ENCLOSED _____
Please pay in U.S. funds only

☐ Check ☐ Money Order ☐ Visa ☐ Mastercard ☐ Discover

Card # _____ Exp. date _____

Signature _____

Complete and mail to:
Hunter House Inc., Publishers
PO Box 2914, Alameda CA 94501-0914
Website: www.hunterhouse.com
Orders: (800) 266-5592 or email: ordering@hunterhouse.com
Phone (510) 865-5282 Fax (510) 865-4295

WMS-R4 8/2000